The Ultimate
CHEST FREEZER
COLD PLUNGE
DIY GUIDE

John Richter

The Ultimate Chest Freezer Cold Plunge DIY Guide

For more information, email: ColdPlunge@JohnRichter.com

http://www.ChestFreezerColdPlunge.com

FOURTH EDITION v.4.7 (October 14, 2020)

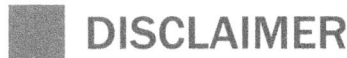
DISCLAIMER

"People who blame others are the cause of all of our problems."
Swami Beyondananda

This guide is provided for entertainment purposes only. Modifying a chest freezer can be dangerous and may result in permanent or irreparable damage. Using an appliance in a way that is not intended by the manufacturer may result in injury or death, so be careful. Use common sense and caution.

ALWAYS UNPLUG YOUR CHEST FREEZER BEFORE GETTING IN!

This guide provides information from the author's views, personal experience, research, and reports from others and is correct to the best of the author's knowledge. No warranties, representations, or guarantees are made about the effectiveness or safety of the information herein.

All information is provided "as is," and might be incomplete, inaccurate, or may not work with your materials, or specific model of chest freezer. By reading or applying any information in this guide, you accept 100% responsibility for your actions and accept the full risk of implementing any of the information herein.

By reading this guide or applying any of the information herein, you fully release the author, his business, family, and his estate of all liability.

The author is not a certified or qualified engineer, builder, manufacturer, sanitation expert, plumber, chemist, or tradesman. If you have any concerns, questions or doubts about applying any of the ideas in this guide, or your skills to do so, consult an appropriately qualified or licensed expert.

Modifying your chest freezer voids the manufacturer's warranty.

The author makes no claims of health benefits or cures. Always consult a doctor or qualified health care practitioner before starting a cold-water immersion practice. Know your limits and be safe.

If all that did not scare you off, keep reading!

WEIGHTS, MEASURES, TEMPERATURES, AND CURRENCY

Both Imperial measurements (pounds, gallons, inches, and Fahrenheit) and Metrics (kilograms, liters, centimeters, and Celsius) are included to benefit a global audience.

Some conversions are rounded up. Double-check my math and your measurements before using any given numbers.

All prices are provided in US Dollars and are current as of the publication of this guide. Prices may be substantially different in your part of the world.

Products mentioned may not be available in all parts of the world. Product substitutes are mentioned when they are known to be of good quality.

 ## PRODUCT COMPATIBILITY IN DIFFERENT COUNTRIES

Ordering appliances and electrical items in your country of origin will ensure compatibility with local power requirements and electrical plugs. When that is not possible, you *might* be able to use a step-down transformer and/or adapter to get a US-made product to work in your county. Use caution!

 ## STATEMENT OF FINANCIAL ARRANGEMENTS

At the time of publication, I have some affiliate or financial arrangements with the manufacturers and retailers of the products mentioned or recommended. If you would like to support ongoing research and updates, please visit the website ChestFreezerColdPlunge.com and purchase products using the links provided.

Use your own best judgment before buying or using any product.

I will never endorse or recommend a product unless I have either used it myself with good results or have reports from many others who have used it with good results.

ACKNOWLEDGMENTS

The history of how this guide came together goes back many years. However, none of it would have started if it had not been for Wim Hof and his work. I want to acknowledge Wim for his commitment to helping everyone become "Happy, Strong, and Healthy."

Much thanks to Elizabeth Lee, who- when I was desperate to find a better way than hauling ice to regularly get into cold water in Austin, Texas- suggested that I look into converting a chest freezer.

I have tremendous gratitude to my 6-year old daughter, Natalia. Since the inception of this project she has helped in countless ways, from making safety signs while I was building, to counting me down to get into the cold water. She reminds me to be playful and inspires me to be a better person.

I appreciate Davey Roxx and Jo Nathan for editing, and Tara Diversi, Mohamed Saheed, and Cameron Slater for their contributions to the layout and graphic design. This guide is better because of your help and input.

I also want to acknowledge the members of the Chest Freezer Cold Plunge Facebook Group who have shared their experiences about what has worked or not, posted pictures of their setups, and provided feedback, inspiration, and encouragement for this project. I do not want to mention specific names for fear of leaving someone out, but to those of you who post frequently and give in-depth answers to other's questions- thank you, you know who you are!

Finally, I want to express appreciation to everyone who commits to stepping out of their comfort zones, getting into cold water, and making their life better.

OVERVIEW OF KEY TOPICS

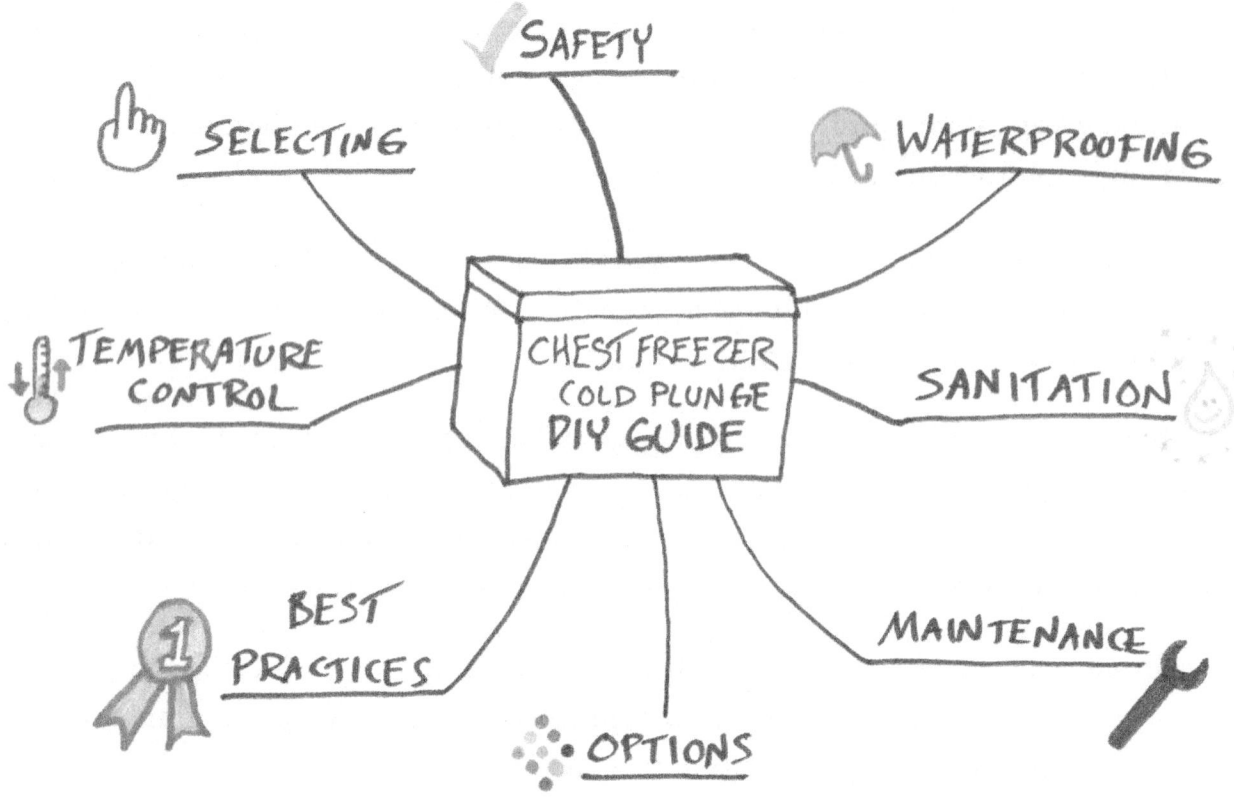

Notes

_____

_____

_____

_____

_____

_____

_____

_____

_____

_____

_____

_____

_____

_____

_____

_____

If you are distressed by anything external,
the pain is not due to the thing itself
but to your own estimate of it;
and this you have the power
to revoke at any moment.

Marcus Aurelius

◼ CONTENTS

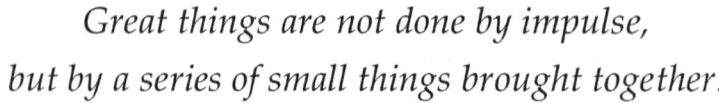

Great things are not done by impulse,
but by a series of small things brought together.

George Eliot

How to Use This Guide

Any Do-It-Yourself (DIY) project is going to involve many variables. Among them are your goals, skillset, and how much you already know.

This guide speaks to the beginner as well as those who may already know the subject.

Because there are so many different ways to set up a chest freezer, there is no one simple shopping list. However, if you make notes as you go along, and use the shopping guide on the next pages, your plan will become clear.

If you are reading the e-book version, you may find it helpful to print the Setup Check List on the following pages and make notes as you go along. Also refer to the Buyer's Guide in the Appendix.

If you are a complete beginner, it is a good idea to read the entire guide. Even the information that you think may not be of interest to you can provide insight into what to do or not do.

If you have already started, skim the table of contents and read the sections that interest you or apply to your system.

Scan the appendices and read any information that applies to your setup.

As mentioned before, if you have questions, post them to the Chest Freezer Cold Plunge Facebook group.

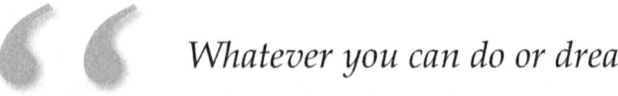 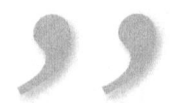

Whatever you can do or dream you can, begin it.

Boldness has genius, power, and magic in it.

Johann Wolfgang von Goethe

Setup Check List

Location
❑ AC Power   ❑ Enough space   ❑ Water-friendly   ❑ Easy to access

Chest Freezer*
Brand: _____   Volume / Size: _____

Inside material: ❑ Painted   ❑ Unpainted

Chest Freezer Length:_____   Width:_____   Depth:_____

Sealants
Brand/Type:_____   Length of Seams: _____   Amount needed: _____

Liners
❑ Not needed   ❑ Pond Liner Size Needed: _____

❑ Custom Liner   ❑ Professionally Installed

Temperature Control
❑ Digital Controller   ❑ Timer   ❑ None- manually unplug/plug in

Water Sanitation
❑ Drain and Clean   ❑ Additives

❑ Pump/Filter   ❑ Chlorine
    Approx. Volume of   ❑ Epsom Salts
    water in chest freezer:_____   ❑ Food Grade H2O2

    Volume x 3 =   ❑ Other:_____
    optimal flow rate / hour: _____

❑ Ozone   ❑ UV Light

Support
❑ Wood shims   ❑ Plastic shims   ❑ Foam mats   ❑ Spray-liner

Compatibility Check
❑ Materials of chest freezer/liner are compatible with my sanitation methods

* Use the Buyer's Check List in Appendix L

Accessories

❑ Long extension cord

❑ Short extension cord (for timer)

❑ GFCI plug or extension cord

❑ Heavy-duty appliance timer

❑ Thermometer

❑ Countdown timer

❑ Garden hose

❑ Shelf or cabinet for devices
(ozone, temp controller, etc.)

❑ Water Pre-filters

❑ Entry/Exit Step

❑ Rubber mat (inside tub)

❑ Bucket

❑ Cleaning Cloth

❑ Fish net

❑ Spa Vacuum

❑ House shoes

Other Materials / Tools

❑ Nitrile / latex gloves (with powder)

❑ Drill

❑ Hole Saw

❑ PVC Plugs

❑ Foam rubber/weather stripping

❑ Wire ties/twist ties

Notes

_____

_____

_____

_____

_____

Introduction

You are most likely reading this because you decided that sitting in cold water can help you, and you would like to find an easier way to make that happen.

You might be brand new to the world of cold-water immersion, or a student of Wim Hof or Dr. Jack Kruze, a professional athlete, or biohacker already using ice baths but looking for a better way.

Buying and hauling ice eats up your time and money. Commercial cold plunges cost thousands of dollars and exceed many people's budgets.

What is the solution?

Convert a chest freezer into a cold plunge!

This guide gives you practical, easy to follow steps, so you can start enjoying the benefits of cold water quickly, safely, and for a long time.

For me, cold water immersion improved my health and a severe case of insomnia. I won't go into more details about that here, but I do include a brief version of my journey of converting a chest freezer into a cold plunge so that you can understand my motivation for writing this guide and why I want to help. Moreover, you will have insight into some of the headaches you can avoid!

MY CHEST FREEZER JOURNEY

I took a weekend course with Wim Hof in Austin, Texas in December of 2013, but had a hard time finding regular access to cold water in our humid subtropical climate. It didn't take too long to grow tired of buying ice and hauling it to my home.

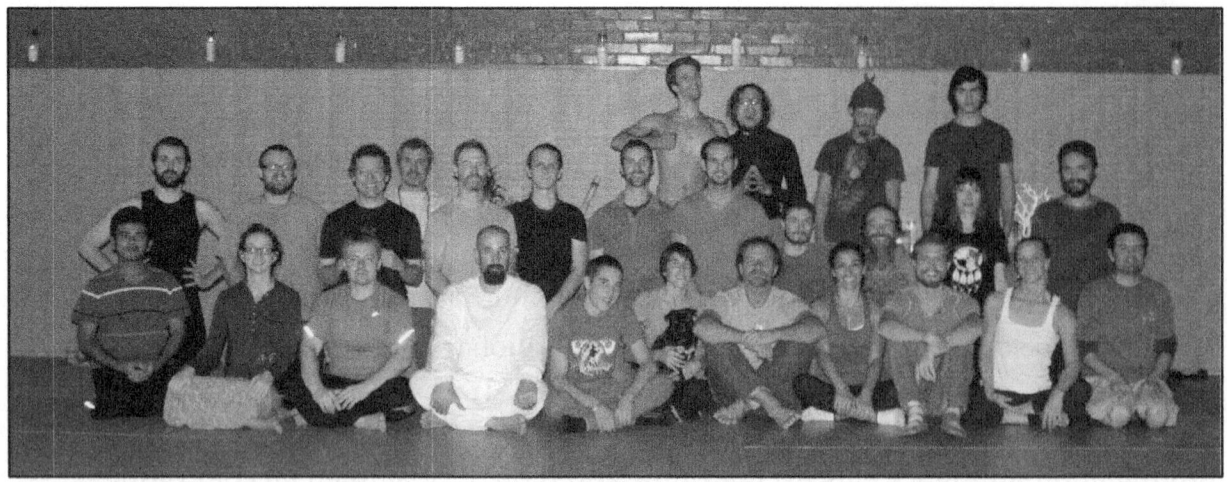

Workshop with Wim Hof, Austin, TX, 2013 (I'm in the back row, third from the left)

When my friend Elizabeth, a certified Wim Hof Method (WHM) trainer, mentioned that some people were using chest freezers to make cold water, I felt a surge of excitement.

However, when I started looking into this process in December of 2016, I found most of the information to be incomplete or contradictory.

About six months later, I bought a new 15 cubic foot (424 L) chest freezer on sale from a local hardware store, brought it home and put it in the garage. I plugged it in, filled it with water, and four days later, on Thursday, July 13, 2017, at 6:55 AM, I climbed in for the first time. I stayed in the 40° F (4.4° C) water for three minutes and felt invigorated. I had created a cold paradise without as much as one cube of ice!

Three days later, my excitement turned to dread when I opened the lid to find rivers of rust seeping out the seams. I unplugged the chest freezer and ran to grab the hose to drain the water. An uneasy feeling in my stomach told me I made an expensive mistake and ruined a new chest freezer.

After the water drained, I placed the chest freezer outside in the sun with the lid open, hoping that it could be salvaged.

That initial failure and feeling of disappointment ignited a spark that evolved into a near obsession for me over the next two years.

Here is some of what went into my process from that point forward: I searched, and researched hundreds of posts on numerous forums, groups, and websites on many topics including:

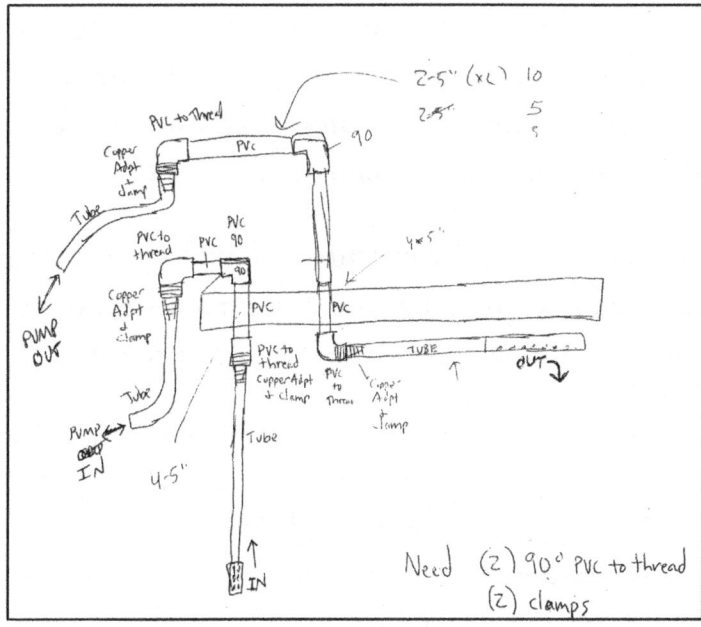

Sketch of an early design

- Appliance repair and construction
- Hot tub and swimming pool construction, repair and maintenance
- Standard chest freezer usage, problems, and maintenance
- Converting chest freezers into keezers (to serve beer on tap)
- Using chest freezers as bait coolers
- Hydroponics and aquaponics
- Aquarium and pond building and maintenance
- Industrial refrigeration and chilling
- Water sanitation
- Plumbing

I flipped through books at the library, talked with people in hardware and appliance stores, appliance repair people, an industrial engineer, and at one point hired a master plumber for a consultation.

For a while, I entertained the idea of building a chest freezer from scratch and talked with people in manufacturing, hot tub companies, industrial chiller reps, and an employee from Underwriter's Laboratory, the global safety certification company that gives products a stamp of approval.

After two years, I went through four significant setups with several smaller changes and tweaks along the way. I spent a little more than $3,500 on different ideas and put blood, sweat, and tears into this project.

Over its first two years of life, my chest freezer setup included:

- Four different types of seals
- Two liners
- External and internal aquarium pumps
- Two different ozone generators
- Removing the lid
- Drilling holes in the lid
- Drilling holes in the floor
- Patching the holes in the floor
- External hot tub pumps and filters with 14' of plumbing
- Building an elevated deck to accommodate the plumbing
- Accidentally scraping off the paint
- Accidentally gouging the internal metal wall
- Stripping the interior paint
- Removing rust from the exposed walls
- Preparing the inside for a spray liner
- Removing and replacing the molding
- Other unexpected fun

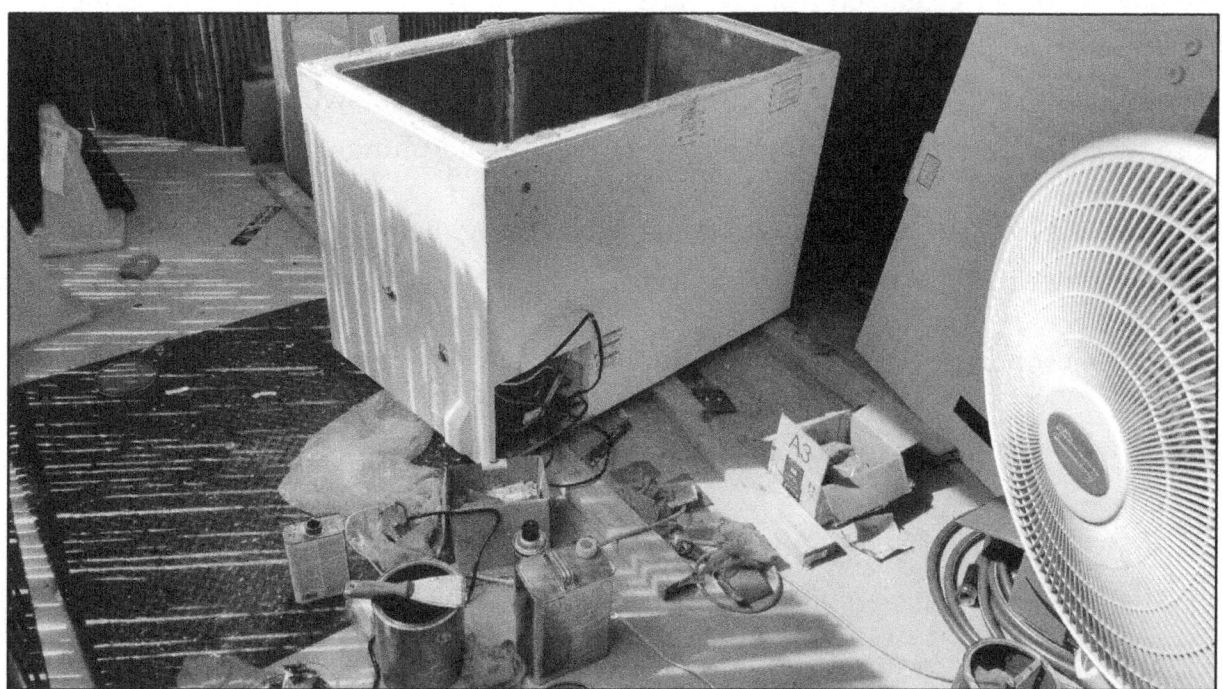

Work in progress

Researching, figuring things out, and experimenting with my chest freezer provided a wealth of information - mostly on what to avoid.

I started the Facebook Group Chest Freezer group in September of 2018 intending to find like-minded people who could share what we learned, mistakes to avoid and celebrate our wins. A little more than a year later there were over 3,900 members from more than 84 countries. There have been hundreds of posts and reports about what works and what doesn't.

I have learned a lot from people's experiences (good and bad), and appreciate their contributions and willingness to help one another. I am also reminded that we can be more connected by what we share in common than divided by our differences.

Fortunately, you can benefit from this collective knowledge on what to do and what mistakes to avoid. This guide will save you time, money, and frustration and provides the best of what I know to tell someone who is starting at the beginning. These are the options I would consider if I had to start over.

That said, my knowledge and expertise are limited. I'm not a plumber, engineer, or chemist and have no formal training in this subject.

I do have knowledge gained from research, practical experience, and the benefit of curating and sorting through a wealth of knowledge from the experience of many others who have dealt with similar problems in hot tubs and swimming pools, and those who have converted their chest freezer into a cold plunge.

As much as I love to research, my passion for teaching, helping people, and making a difference brings me an even greater sense of joy and fulfillment.

Before we jump in, there are a few more things to cover.

WHERE TO START AND HOW TO USE THIS GUIDE

"If you don't know where you are going,
you'll end up someplace else."

Yogi Berra

This guide includes useful and practical information on various ways to convert a chest freezer into a cold plunge. You'll learn best practices, pitfalls to avoid, and practical tips on how to use and maintain your cold plunge.

If you know what you want to do, you can skip ahead to the sections that are of interest. However, you might find it useful to read through other sections because you might learn something that could apply to your setup, inspire a creative idea, or help you plan for things to add in the future.

Although it is beyond the scope of this guide, a little bit of information is included about the benefits of cold water and cold-water training.

If you are new to cold water training, I urge you to attend a workshop with Wim Hof or one of his certified instructors or take one of his online programs. The Wim Hof Method goes beyond getting into cold water. His programs include other practices that help people become "Happy, Healthy, and Strong." I enthusiastically recommend his online and live courses.

VOIDING YOUR WARRANTY

The Disclaimer mentioned this, but in case you didn't read it, here it is again.

These actions void your chest freezer warranty:

- Sealing the seams
- Painting or coating the inside or outside
- Drilling or cutting holes in the walls, floor, or lid
- Filling it with water

If you feel nervous about voiding your warranty, this may be a good exercise in letting go. Enjoy it!

 ## HOW TO GET HELP AND SUPPORT

If you get stuck, have questions, or want to discuss a new option, visit the Chest Freezer Cold Plunge Facebook Group. We welcome questions and updates about your progress. Provide details about the setup you have chosen, what works, and what doesn't work.

I am also available for private consulting about your chest freezer project. See my website for details.

I encourage you to post pictures and video of your cold tub system and you and your family enjoying it.

I'm looking forward to hearing about your setup and experience with your *Chest Freezer Cold Tub*.

Sincerely,

John Richter

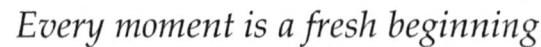

Every moment is a fresh beginning.

T.S. Eliot

Chapter 1: Safety

While cold water can provide tremendous health benefits, it can also cause injury or death. Chest freezers are not designed to hold water. Pouring water into a device that plugs into an electrical outlet may create a risk of electrocution.

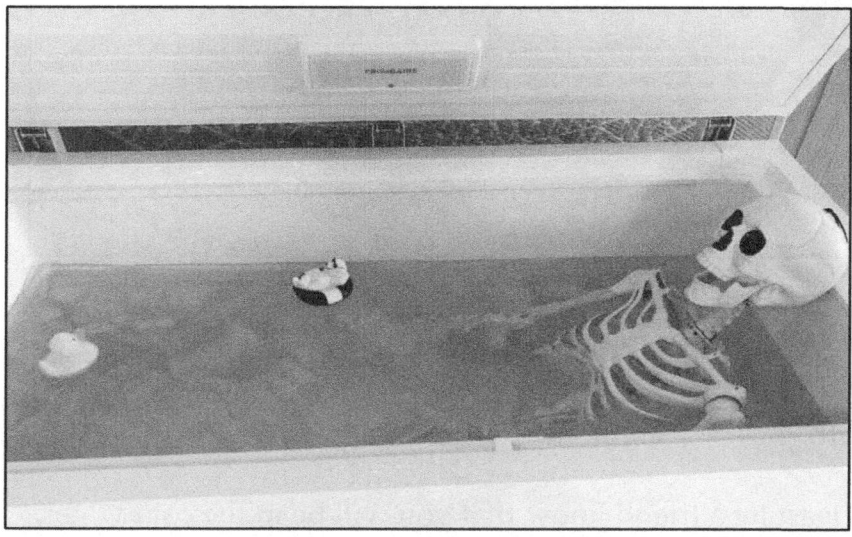

Photo couresy of Troy Delaney, Jacksonville,

 ## ALWAYS UNPLUG!

Always unplug your chest freezer before you get in!

Always unplug pumps, timers, temperature controllers, ozone generators, UV lights, and any other electrical components that are part of your system.

Do not use headphones, phones, tablets, or other electrical devices when you are in your chest freezer. This message repeats throughout this guide.

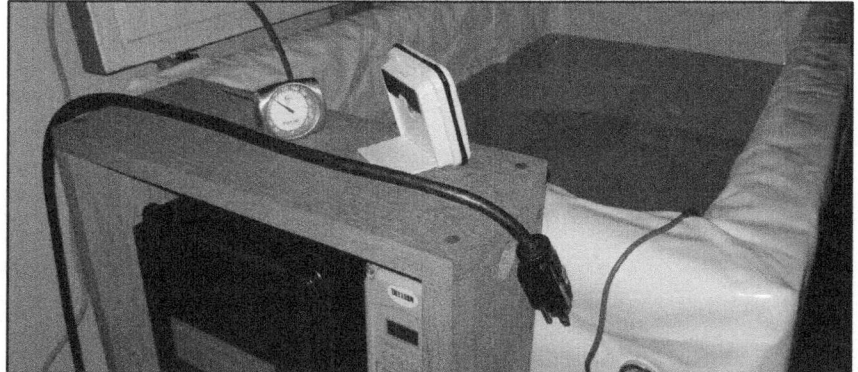

Unplug your chest freezer before getting in

USE THE BUDDY SYSTEM!

Whenever you get into cold water, always have a friend nearby. Even the most experienced, healthiest, and strongest among us can have an off day. Having

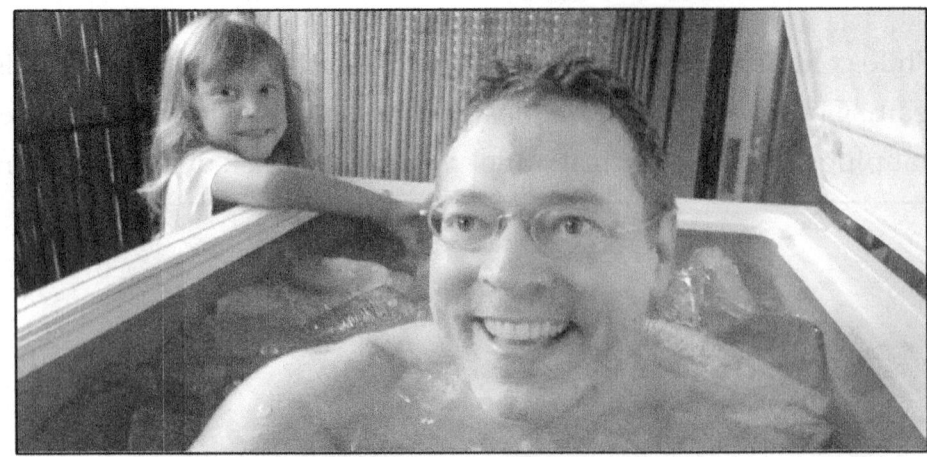

My daughter, Natalia, loves to count me down to get in

a buddy nearby can make the difference between an annoyance and an injury, or even, between life and death.

If you must train alone, at least let a friend know that you will be in the cold water, and let them know you will check-in after you have finished. Set up a plan that if your friend doesn't hear from you, they will call emergency services. That might sound dramatic, but it's better to be safe than sorry.

 ## WHAT IF THE LID CLOSES WHILE YOU ARE INSIDE?

Some people feel concerned about the lid closing while they sit inside the chest freezer. In the US, before 1956, refrigerators and freezers automatically locked when closed. The doors on models made after that date were required by law to open from the inside. Modern freezers are safer now than vintage models, but there are still some things to keep in mind.

Modern chest freezers have strong hinges that hold the lid open until you decide to close it.

If you still feel nervous about the lid closing, there are a few things to do and consider:

1. Look for a chest freezer that cannot lock accidentally.

The Whirlpool models have the lock *below* the lid which requires the key (and thus the latch inside) to be turned *upward* to lock the chest freezer. The only way for it to lock accidentally would be to defy gravity.

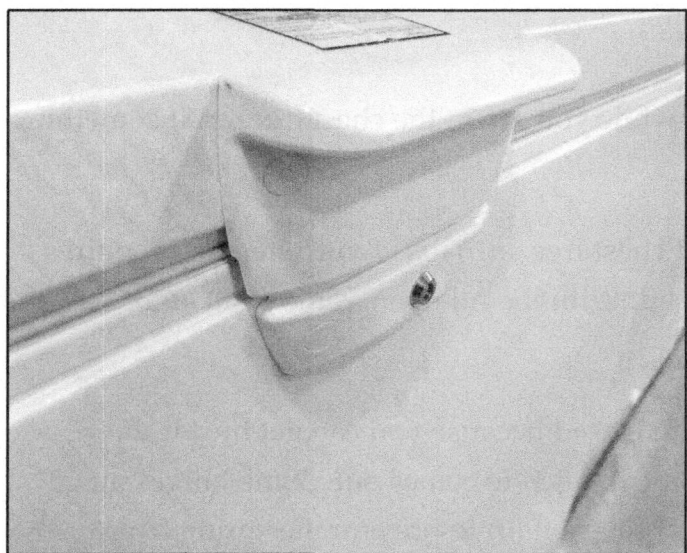

Whirlpool handle and lock

Frigidaire models have a lock on the lid handle, but the key must be pressed inward to push the lock backward before it turns to engage the latch, making it impossible to lock by accident.

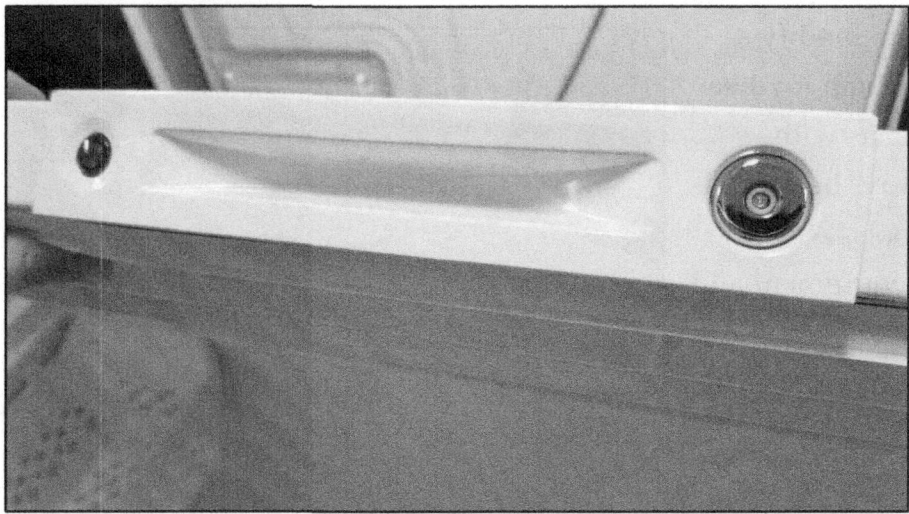

Frigidaire handle and lock

2. For most people, if the lid falls while you are sitting in the chest freezer, your head will stop it from closing all the way. This might result in an unpleasant hit but is unlikely to knock you out.

3. Fold or roll up your towel and place it on the front wall or over the front corner of your chest freezer. If the lid falls while you are doing a head dunk, the towel will prevent the lid from closing all the way.

4. Have a trusted friend stand nearby while you are in the chest freezer. If something goes wrong, they are there to help.

5. Remove the hinges from the lid and chest freezer. This is a big step and requires extra work to remove and replace the lid. With the lid open, remove all eight screws from each hinge.

Do NOT remove the hinges with the lid closed because you can get hurt if the springs in the hinges pop open when the last screw comes out. Some hinges may have a small opening to insert an object (like a nail) to prevent the spring from popping open and hurting you. Be VERY careful when removing hinges!

If you remove the hinges, place a weight on the closed lid to help it seal.

 WORK ZONE

There are many ways to modify a chest freezer. Some of them involve power tools and products with strong chemicals. Always be careful when working with tools. Wear the recommended safety equipment and be sure to use the tools as recommended. If you are not comfortable using specific tools, enroll a handy friend to help.

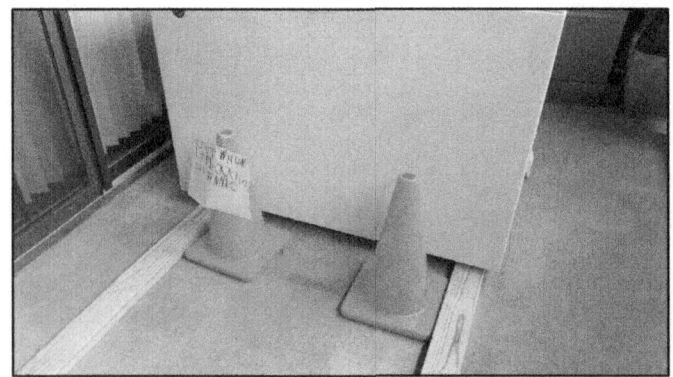

Safety cones with a sign made by my 4-year old

When working with chemicals, be sure your area is well ventilated and wear a respirator and gloves. Some people are OK with latex, but I find that they rip easily. I prefer thicker mechanics gloves.

GET TRAINING

What do world-class athletes, entrepreneurs, and CEO's all have in common? Most have coaches or mentors who help them become their best and avoid pitfalls. The Introduction mentioned getting training, but the idea is worth repeating.

A small, but unfortunately growing number of new people have hurt themselves by staying in very cold water much longer than they should have. What do they all have in common? They had no idea what they were doing.

There are number of ways to learn how to be safe in cold water:
- Attend a Wim Hof workshop (live or online)
- Hire a certified Wim Hof trainer
- Join a group and ask a lot of questions. Check out the Facebook groups for the Wim Hof Method and Dr. Jack Kruse.

What is the best training? In my opinion, the Wim Hof Method! It's best to take a workshop from a certified instructor. You can find instructors on this website: www.wimhofmethod.com/instructors

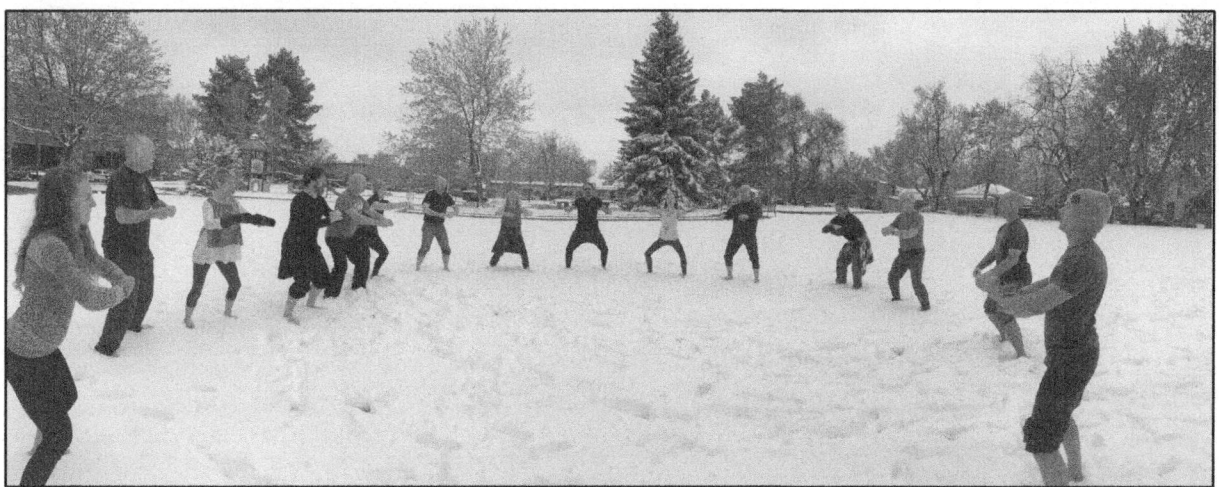

Wim Hof Fundamentals Course in Denver, Colorado with Elizabeth Lee, Level 3 certified WHM instructor

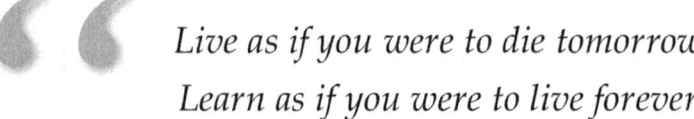

Live as if you were to die tomorrow.
Learn as if you were to live forever.

Mahatma Gandhi

Chapter 2: Questions to Ask Before You Start Shopping

"There are hundreds of ways to kneel and kiss the ground."

Rumi

 WHAT DO YOU WANT?

Each person has different values, resources, and goals. Here are a few things to consider:

- What is your budget for this project?

- Are you looking for a short-term or long-term solution?

- How much time are you willing to spend setting it up?

- Can you make a regular commitment to maintenance?

- How much or how little maintenance are you willing to do?

- How often do you plan to use your cold tub?

- Do you prefer to keep things simple, or do you love hacking, tinkering, and building things?

Keep this in mind: it's better to get started with something than to take too much time analyzing and planning. This guide removes a significant number of unknowns from the process, and it is up to you to take action!

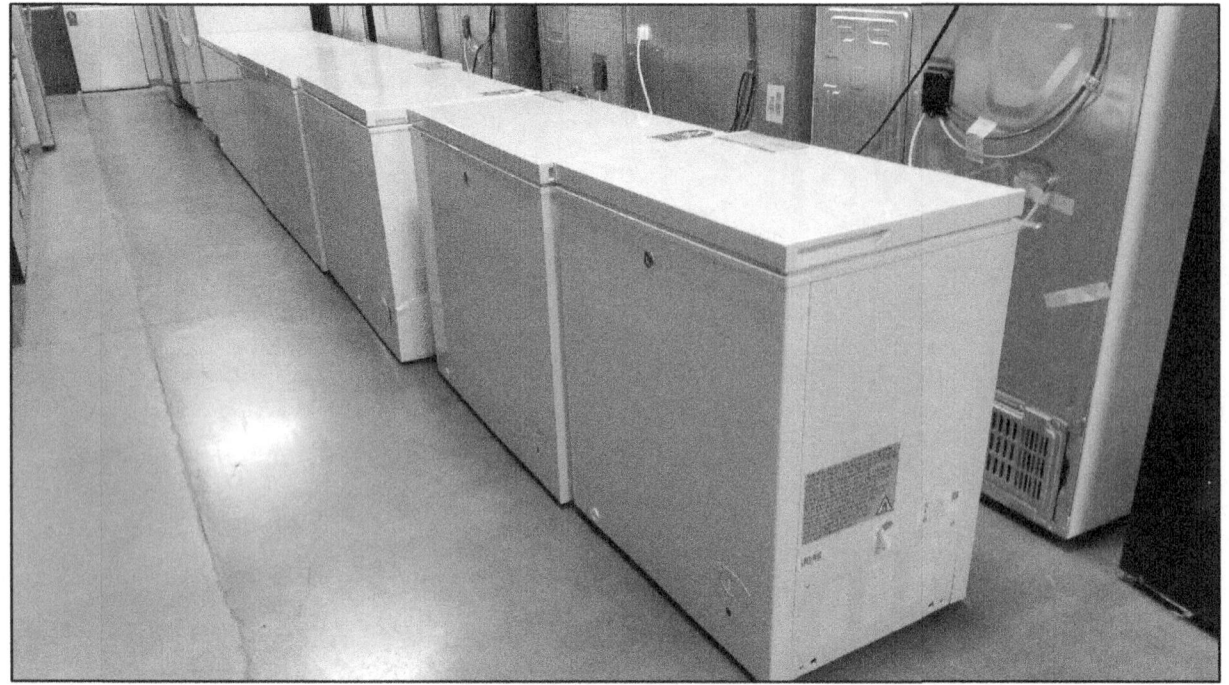

At the appliance store

WHERE WILL YOU PUT YOUR CHEST FREEZER?

Before you start shopping for a chest freezer, think about where you can place it. Measure your space to make sure it works for your freezer.

Avoid exposure to direct sunlight, rain, hail, snow, dust, bugs, rodents, or other animals.

THINGS TO CONSIDER

- Will your chest freezer fit through the door?

- Is there a power outlet nearby?

- Is there anything close by that is flammable or susceptible to heat? The outside walls of the chest freezer can get very hot.

- Is there anything nearby that could be damaged by splashing, leaking, or pooling water?

- Do you have enough space to leave a few inches around the sides and back for ventilation? Three inches (8 cm) is recommended.

- Is there enough space behind and above for the lid to open?

- Do you have enough room to safely and quickly get in and out of the chest freezer from the front?

- Is there any risk of theft?

- Do you have enough room for optional components such as an ozone generator, extension cords, or temperature controller?

■ Convenience

An important question to ask is, "How convenient and easy will it be for me to get to the freezer each time I want to use it?"

If you have to go through a bunch of doors, walk across a large yard, remove a padlock, or jump through other hoops, you may be less inclined to use your cold plunge, especially on those days where feel some resistance.

Wherever you decide to put it, make sure that it is easy to access.

■ Ambient Temperature & Climate

Most chest freezers are designed to be inside a climate-controlled home. Unless you have plenty of space (or happen to be a bachelor), setting it up inside can be problematic, and will likely cause serious Feng shui issues.

Many people keep them in a garage.

Some manufacturers make chest freezers designed to work in a garage. These freezers are more efficient and may last longer, but they can cost as much as 30% more than basic models.

The ambient temperature can impact how well your freezer works. Most freezer user guides say to keep it in a room between 50° - 90° F (10° - 32.2° C). These guidelines consider food safety and optimal temperature range for the refrigerant.

Cooler ambient air helps your chest freezer work less. However, problems can arise when it gets too cold.

1. Frost can build up on the components as well as on the insulation beneath the exterior walls. When it gets warm outside, the frost thaws, producing moisture that can damage the insulation and cause the freezer to run the compressor more often. It can also rust the walls from the inside out.

2. The viscosity of the oils used to lubricate moving parts may be affected, which can cause them to break down.

3. Seals and gaskets may crack.

Scorching ambient temperatures and high humidity cause the compressor to run more often, reducing the life of your freezer.

If you live near the coast and put your chest freezer outside, corrosion will become an issue.

If your chest freezer is outside, strong winds can catch an open lid and damage or break the hinges, preventing the lid from sealing correctly, or staying open on its own. An improper seal can allow warm air, dust, or critters to get inside.

Here are a few places people have put their chest freezer cold plunge:

- Inside their home
- Garage
- Covered or enclosed porch or patio
- Covered outdoor area
- Shed
- Outside, fully exposed (not recommended)

Real World Setup

The below pictures show a delightful setup from Catherine P. who lives in the UK. She is using her chest freezer cold plunge to train for a swim in the Antarctica. She created an inviting, magical space for her setup.

It is inside of a shed which has been decorated with lights, motivational signs, and made to feel comfortable and inviting. It looks like a great place to hang out!

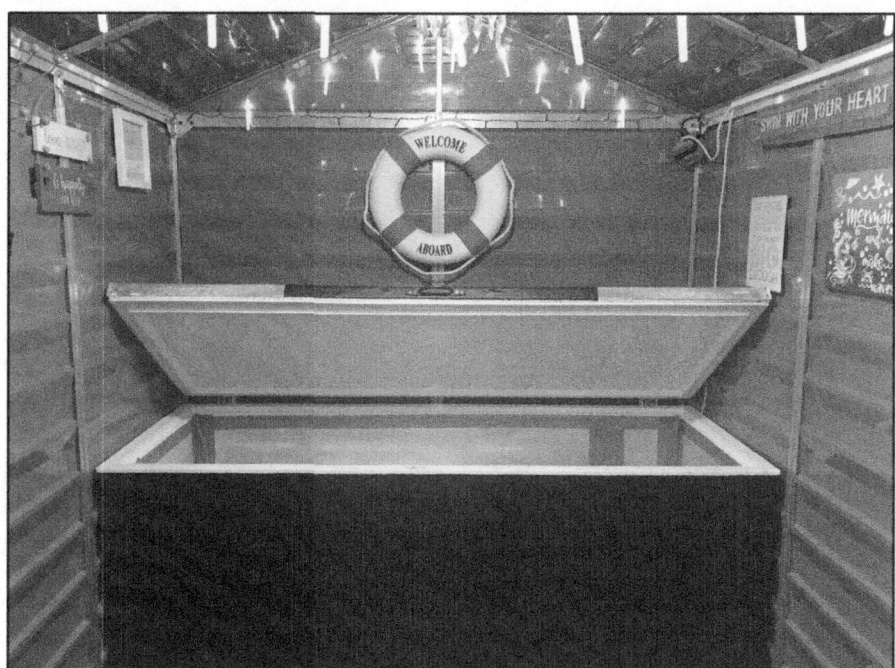

Catherine's Ice Palace

"*The people who get on in this world*

are the people who get up and

look for the circumstances they want

and if they can't find them, make them."

George Bernard Shaw

Chapter 3: Selecting the Best Chest Freezer

There are a few things to consider when purchasing a chest freezer. This section covers the most common concerns and can help you make the best selection for your needs. Because everyone has different goals and budgets, there is no single "best" chest freezer system.

 ## 1. WHAT IS MY PLAN?

Before you buy your chest freezer, figure out as many details as possible.

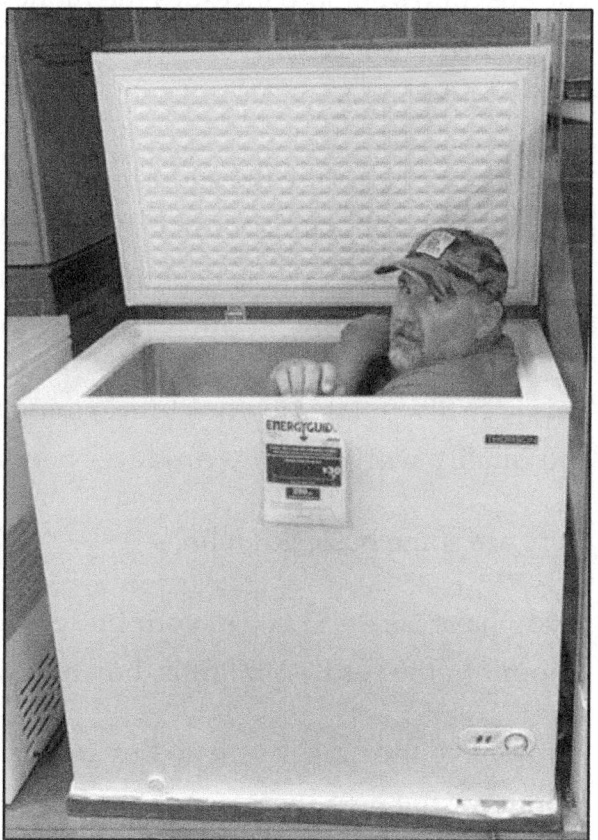

- How do you plan to seal it?

- How do you want to sanitize the water?

- Do you plan to use it long term or short term?

- What is your budget?

Answering as many questions as you can before you buy your chest freezer helps prevent costly mistakes. For example, let's say that you want to install an expensive, very nice spray liner and use ozone to sanitize your water. If you know in advance that ozone deteriorates the material in that spray liner, you can avoid making an expensive mistake.

Mick P. "test driving" chest freezers in South Carolina, USA

2. NEW OR USED?

Is it better to buy a new or used chest freezer? The main thing to consider when answering this question is your budget and tolerance for things to go wrong.

TIP

Use the Inspection Check List for Buying a Chest Freezer in Appendix L.

Most people think about their budget as how much money they have or can set aside to make a purchase. The amount of dollars paid for an item is known as your *cost to buy*.

However, what most people do not consider is the *cost of ownership* over time. The cost of ownership includes the money spent on parts and other products used for maintenance, repairs, and eventual replacement. I also like to consider the cost and value of my time.

There are cases where the short-term cost of buying something is most important. However, over the long term, it almost always ends up being less expensive to spend more money in the beginning to buy the highest quality of materials. Why? Because high-quality products tend to outlast those of lower quality.

This idea also relates to your time. Going slow and focusing your attention on detail and quality workmanship produces better results than rushing.

Here are some basic guidelines:

If you have $600 - $1,500 in your budget now for a complete system, or can save that amount in the next 4-6 months, buy a new chest freezer.

If you have the money now to buy a new chest freezer and can save $100 - $200 a month for the next several months, buy a new freezer now and add to your system as you can.

If you have less than $200 - $300 to spend right now, and it will take more than six to twelve months to save enough to buy a new one, a used chest freezer is a good way to start. Set aside money each month for repairs or to eventually buy a new chest freezer. And mentally prepare yourself to not be attached if it stops working.

■ Used Chest Freezers

Used chest freezers have a higher risk of breaking down. You must be willing to risk investing time and effort to set up your chest freezer and be prepared to fix it if it breaks.

Older chest freezers may use more electricity, either because they have larger, less efficient components or because they are wearing out.

Real World Setup

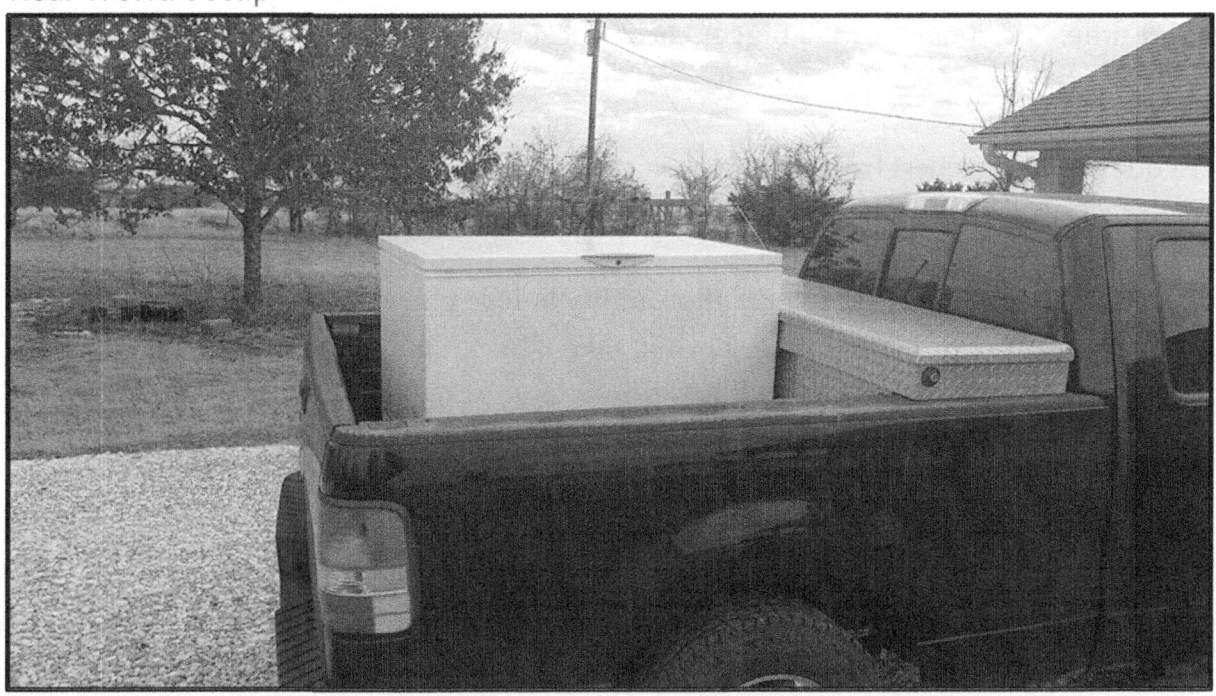

Picking up a used chest freezer, David Wheeler, Waco TX

Brand/Size: Frigidaire 15-cu. ft. (424 L)

Date Set Up: December 2018

Seams: Sealed with Maine Sealant

Water Sanitation: MarineLand aquarium pump/filter, JED Ozone Generator

Comments: Noticed white residue floating in the water after a month, but has not been a problem since then (about 7 months later).

If you do buy a used chest freezer, ask the owner to plug it in and select the coldest setting at least one day before you arrive. Bring a thermometer.

Place it on the compressor compartment inside the freezer and close the lid. Wait about a minute and check your thermometer.

Ideally, the temperature should be pretty close to 0° F (-18° C). If it is much warmer than that, find another chest freezer.

Be friendly and ask why they are selling the chest freezer and how old it is. If it is more than five or 10 years old, you might want to pass. It is possible to find used chest freezers that are less than a year or two old. Sometimes people need them for a short time, and others want a bigger chest freezer with more room.

 New Chest Freezers

If you buy a new chest freezer, there are several options to consider. A few of these include brand, size, and the type of material used for the inside walls and floor.

Always inspect your chest freezer thoroughly before you start converting it into a cold plunge. If you find anything wrong, take it back for an exchange.

As with used chest freezers, plug it in and put it on the coldest setting and place a thermometer inside. Within 12 – 24 hours the temperature inside should be close to 0° F (-18° C). If it is not, exchange it for another unit.

Chest freezers can be subject to much abuse in stores, warehouses, and during shipping. Keep your receipt. Be sure your seller offers an easy return policy. If you bought it via mail or had it shipped, be sure that return and replacement shipping is covered if there is a problem.

If you find any problems, call the retailer and arrange for a return/replacement. Most retailers are not super knowledgeable about the chest freezers they sell. If you have concerns about how it works, call the phone number for the manufacturer's customer service line. It should be in the instruction manual or user guide.

3. WHAT IS THE BEST BRAND?

There are only a handful of manufacturers that make chest freezers. They get labeled with different brand names depending upon where you live in the world. Most major brands should be fine. Avoid chest freezers that are knock-off brands or made by obscure companies whose names you've never heard. Search Consumer Reports and reviews before you decide.

If possible, buy and pick up your chest freezer from a local store. That reduces the chance of damage during delivery. If your car is not large enough to hold the chest freezer, find a friend with a truck or trailer or pay for the delivery.

For our purpose, I do not believe that there is a significant difference between the major brands of chest freezers.

See Appendix D for a list of a few major chest freezer brands in different countries.

4. WHAT SIZE DO I NEED?

What is the best size chest freezer for you to use? One that is comfortable to sit in, easy to climb in and out of, fits into your space, and feels joyful to use. Avoid a freezer if you have to squeeze or bend to fit, or feel claustrophobic while inside.

Keep in mind that unlike hot tubs, we typically only sit in our cold plunges for a few minutes at a time. Some people keep their water temperature around 55°F (12° C) and prefer lounging for 30-45 minutes.

However, most people do not use their cold plunge for relaxing, socializing, or hanging out. Because of that, you don't need an overly large chest freezer.

It is equally important to make sure your chest freezer is not too small. For safety, you should be able to easily and quickly get into and out of your chest freezer. When sitting inside, if your body presses against the walls, get the next larger size.

I have seen many pictures and videos of people who sit in cold water with good intentions but only made a partial commitment. What do I mean by that? They were only in the water up to their waist, belly, or chest.

Sometimes this was because they chose to do it that way. However, in many cases, it was because their container was too small.

For most people with a height under 5′ 10″ (17 7 cm), and weight less than 200 lbs. (90 kg), a 15 cubic foot (300 L) chest freezer works fine.

If you are taller than 6′ (183 cm), or weigh more than 250 lbs. (113 kg), consider buying a 21+ cubic foot (400+ L) chest freezer. Larger chest freezers, while not much taller or deeper than the smaller models, are wider and have more room to stretch out your legs.

TIP

I don't have any scientific data to back this up, but in my personal experience, there's something vastly different and better (but initially scarier) about immersing yourself in cold water so that it covers your shoulders.

I have a strong hunch that the beneficial physiological response increases when you have more of your body submerged.

In the three pictures I took sitting in different sized chest freezers, my back is against the side wall with my feet extended as far as possible along the floor.

I wasn't consciously thinking about it at the time, but looking at the pictures afterward, I found it interesting how the expression on my face changed as the chest freezer's size increased.

Keep in mind that larger chest freezers consume more power and require more water to fill. They also need larger accessories like liners or circulation pumps. The difference is not significant, however, and I would not use that reason alone to buy a smaller sized freezer.

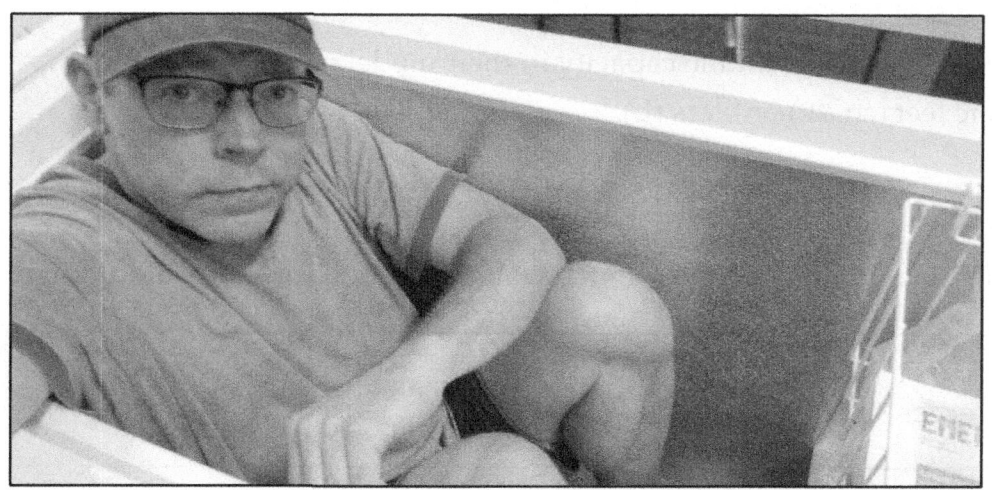

7.8 cubic feet- cramped

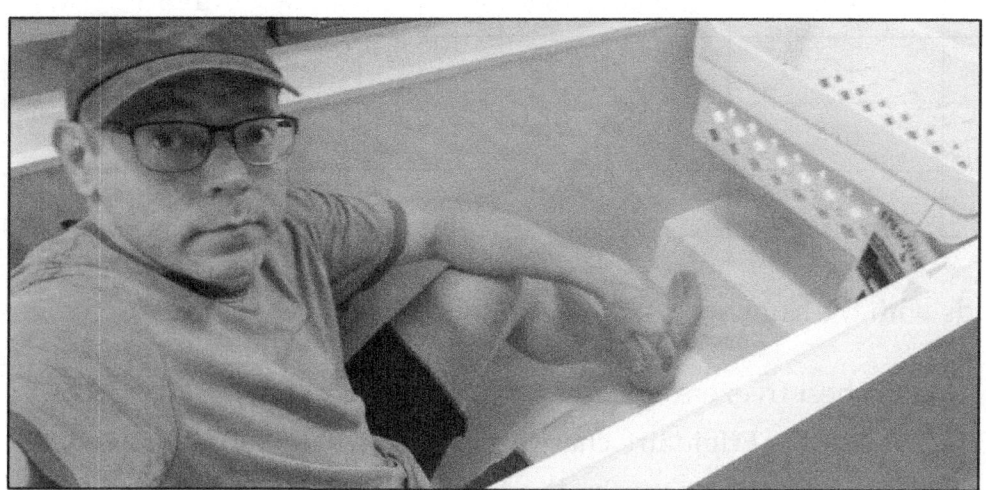

15 cubic feet- better

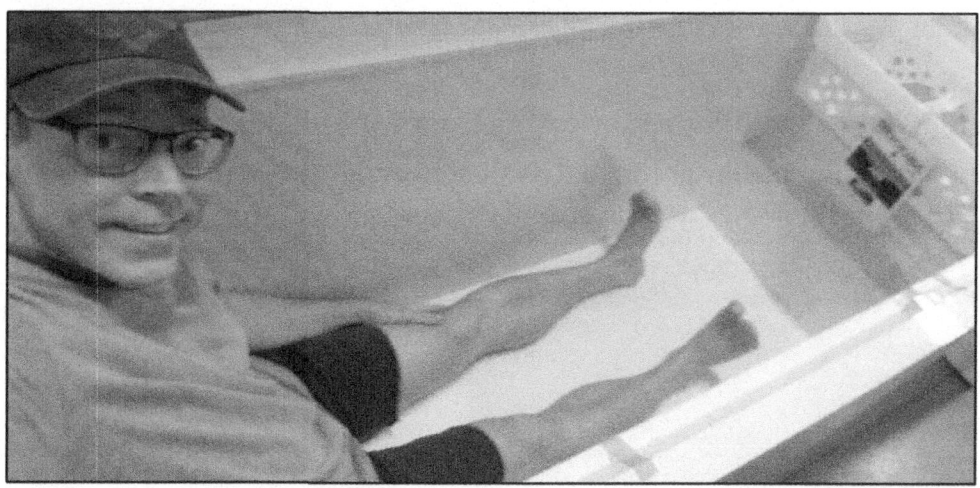

19.8 cubic feet- more than enough space

◼ Size and Volume of Water

Chest freezers usually have a volume capacity in their model name. The capacity is described in cubic feet (cu. ft.) or liters (L).

The difference from one size to the next is significant.

Here are typical sized options with how much water is needed for your cold plunge.

Chest Freezer Size		Approximate Volume of Water for Cold Plunge	
Cubic Feet	Liters	Gallons	Liters
7.0	198	39	148
14.8	419	70	265
21.7	614	108	408
25.0	708	179	678

In different brands with the same volume, there can be differences in measurements.

For example, Frigidaire chest freezers are 9 inches wider than Whirlpool, but the whirlpools are 3 inches deeper. Frigidaire chest freezers also have more than twice as much space taken up inside the freezer by the cover over the compressor compartment.

◼ Compressor Compartments

The next two pictures show the compressor covers from two different 15 cubic foot chest freezers. The Frigidaire cover, going across the entire width, takes up more than twice the space of the Whirlpool cover.

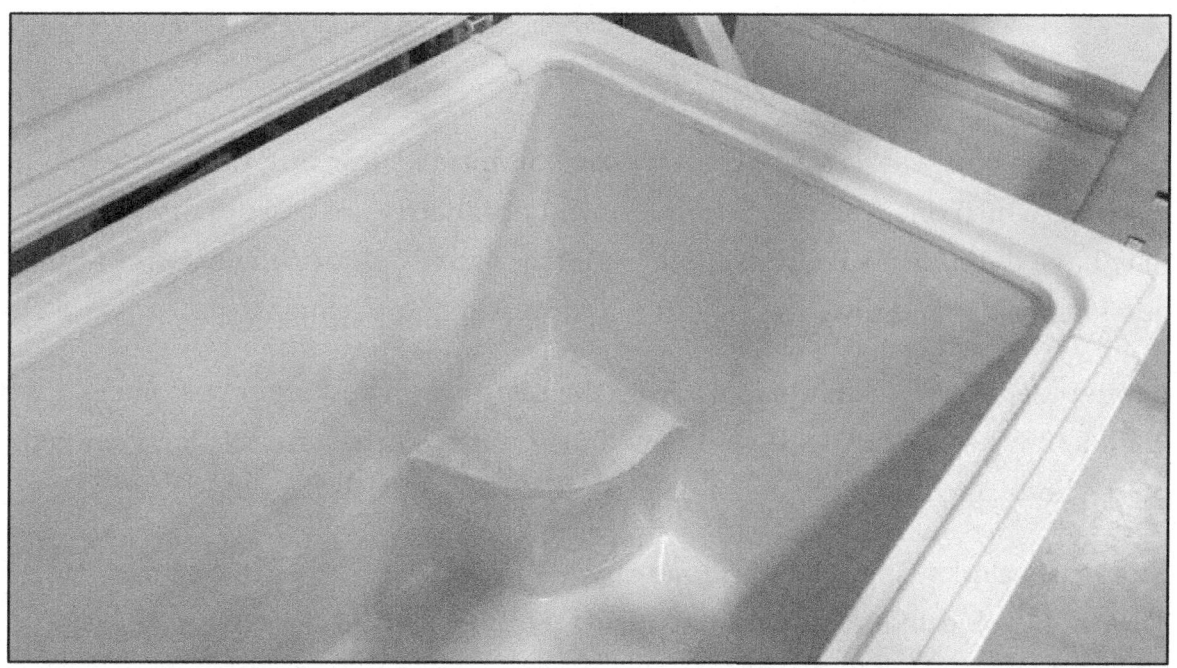

Whirlpool compressor cover

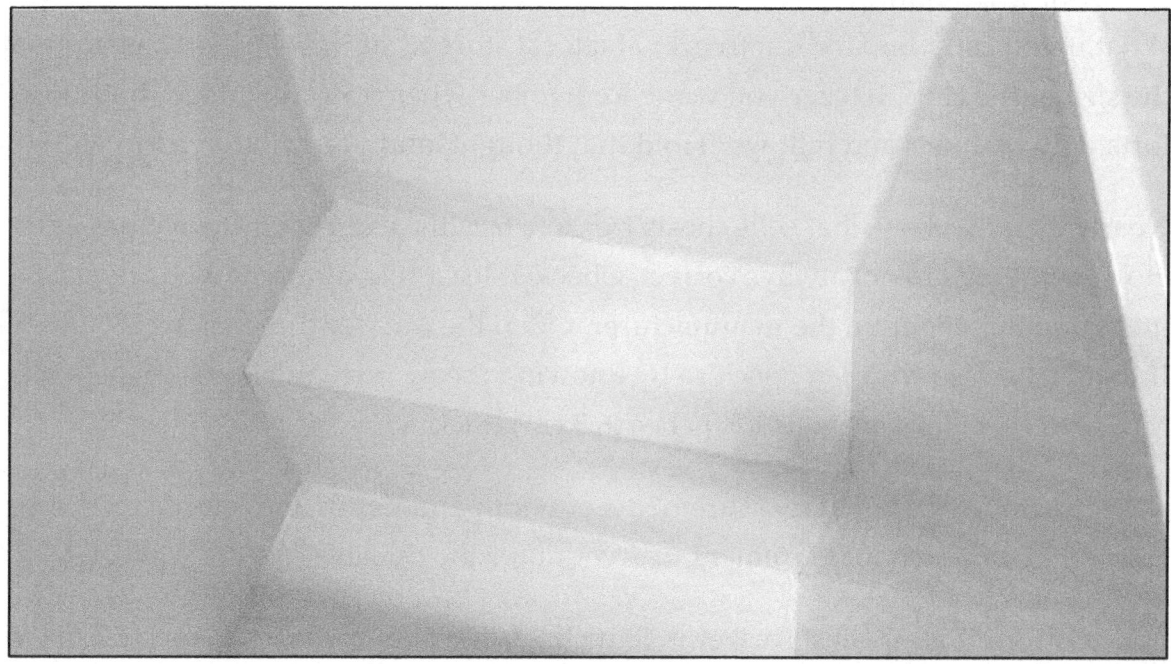

Frigidaire compressor cover

Sitting in Chest Freezers

What is the best way to size a chest freezer? Sit inside a few different models to discover which one feels most comfortable. Local hardware and appliance stores may have them in stock. Bring along a tape measure. Get the dimensions of the outside, inside, and the cover over the compressor compartment.

Be prepared for some funny looks from the salesperson and other customers. If you want to have some fun, let them know that you need a chest freezer large enough to hold a body. Go into more detail quickly, so they don't call the police.

Most sales clerks either left me alone or were fascinated by the cold-plunge project. They never objected to me climbing inside. However, one national retailer had attached transparent plastic sheets over the opening to keep people out.

Use Your Imagination

What if you can't find a chest freezer at a local store to sit in? Mark off a space that is the size of the chest freezer you want. Remember when you were a kid, building forts with blankets and pillows? Hold that thought, and you will have fun with this!

Nearly every website that sells chests freezers lists the external dimensions. However, they are not always correct. Check at least two different websites, including the one from the manufacturer. Often the interior dimensions are missing. If that is the case, you can get close by knowing the average thickness of the walls. Most exterior walls average 2.5 inches (6.3 cm) thick.

Take the known external measurements of width and depth and subtract 5 inches (12.7 cm) from each measurement to account for the thickness of the walls.

For example, if your chest freezer is 48 inches wide and 27 inches deep (122 x 69 cm), subtract the average wall thickness to get 43 x 22 inches (109 x 56 cm).

Be sure to take into account the size of the area that is taken up by the compressor. For example, the cover over the Frigidaire compressor is 8.75 inches (22 cm) wide, so your final marked area would be 34.25 x 22 inches, or (87 x 56 cm).

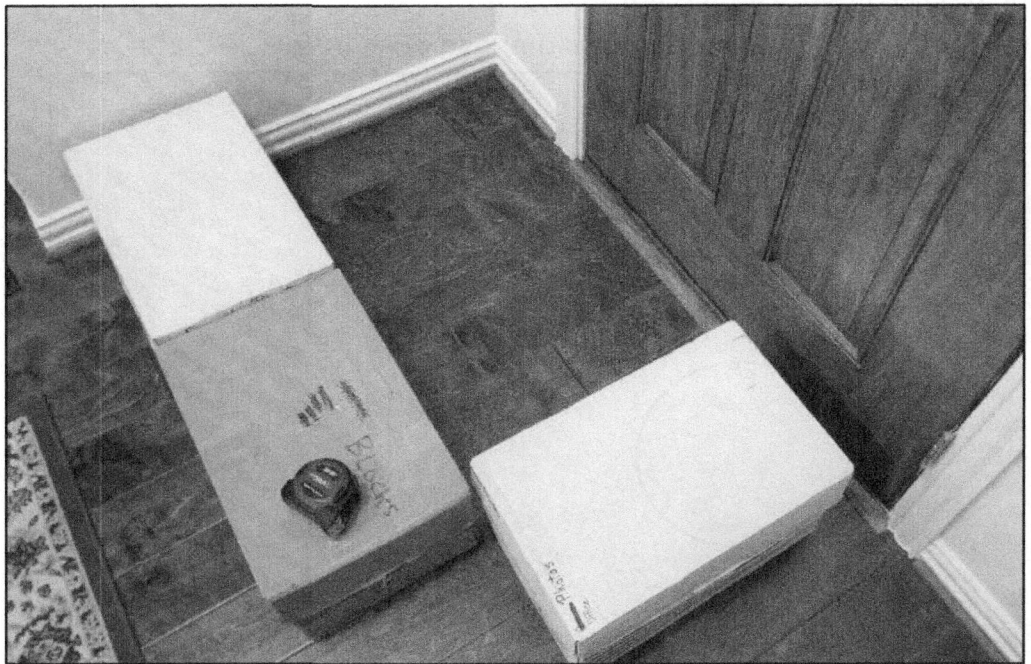

Sizing your imaginary chest freezer

After you know your internal dimensions, use masking tape, cardboard, boxes, or any other items to mark out an area representing the inside of your chest freezer.

Create the area near the corner of a room so you'll have something to lean against.

Sit down inside your marked area. Imagine the walls (or other walls). Is it comfortable, or do you feel squished? If you feel cramped in that space, it's a good idea to get the next larger size.

I am 5'-10" (178 cm) and weigh 175 lbs. (79 kg). While I *can* squeeze into a 7.8-cu. ft. (221 L) chest freezer, it is a tight, uncomfortable fit. I found the 21-cu. ft. (600 L) models to be much larger than I needed. The 15-cu. ft. (400 L) model was perfect.

▮ 5. INSIDE WALLS: PAINTED VS. UNPAINTED

Chest freezers interiors are either painted or unpainted. I used to think that there was not much difference between the two. Now I know better.

Years ago, I bought a small 5-cu. ft. chest freezer for storing extra food. It had bare metal walls, and we used it for about ten months. When we defrosted it to put it up for sale, I discovered a 1" long split in the metal over the floor. We never dropped anything in the freezer, and I wondered if maybe the damage was caused by too much frost buildup or the weight of the items that had been inside.

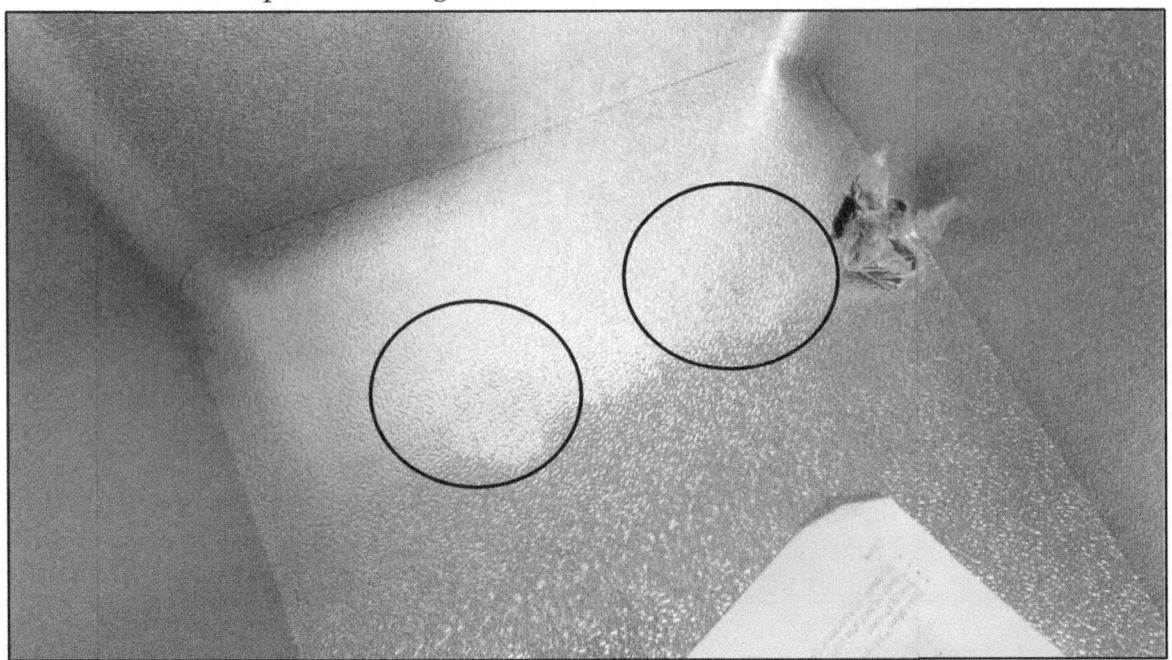

Dents in an aluminum floor

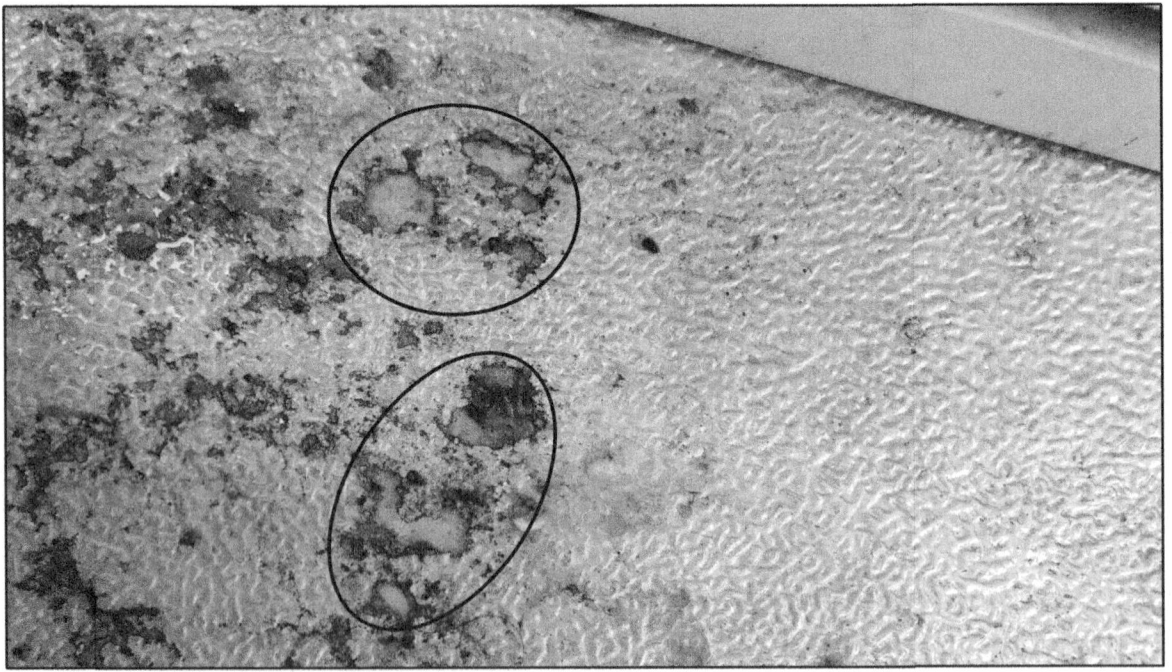

Holes in an aluminum floor exposing the insulation

Years later, after taking pictures of different chest freezers, I noticed that the ones with unpainted walls had many dents.

One unpainted chest freezer that I climbed into, without shoes, had very noticeable impressions where I was standing and sitting. The freezers with painted walls/floors had no apparent dents.

The unpainted walls are constructed from thin aluminum. Painted walls are made of steel (at least in the Whirlpool brand) and coated with an enamel that is baked on at the factory. I also noticed that over the last few years that Frigidaire started using painted walls instead of unpainted in their larger models.

Many people use chest freezers with unpainted walls, and you might have great success doing so. However, I have a hunch that the chest freezers with painted walls last longer because they seem to be stronger and more durable, which is why I recommend them.

If you end up with unpainted inside walls, place a wet area mat on the bottom inside to protect the floor. See Chapter 6: Equipment & Accessories for more information. Definitely use a liner of some kind.

Another issue with bare metal walls is that they can be damaged by salt, chlorine, ozone, and… just water. Aluminum does not rust like other metals; however, it is likely that the chest freezer walls are an aluminum alloy, or contain impurities. Depending on what other metals are present, the water temperature, and the concentration of chemicals, the reaction rate can be longer or shorter.

Salt and chlorine react with aluminum, causing pitting and a whitish residue to form. Different charts state that aluminum and chlorine have either a "C-fair" or "D-severe effect" compatibility.

If you are shopping online, it might be difficult to determine if a particular chest freezer has the painted or bare metal interior. Look at all of the pictures and you will almost always find one of the baskets holding food. Look at the interior wall.

If it is a silver/gray color, or textured, it is bare metal. If it is smooth and white, it has the baked on enamel coating.

6. WHAT TO AVOID

Here are a few features and products that are unnecessary and will either increase your cost, frustration, amount of work needed, or the potential for problems.

- Rollers, casters, or wheels
  (unless they can be removed, but that opens other potential issues)

- Automatic defrost

- Extended warranty

- Ice-cream freezer

- Glass lids that slide open

- Commercial or industrial chest freezers

- Laboratory chest freezers

- Walk-in freezers

At one point, I thought it would be awesome to buy a walk-in freezer. I could have an arctic environment and a cold plunge inside. They cost several thousands of dollars, have special electrical requirements, and can be very expensive to maintain. Maybe one day!

7. TEMPERATURE SETTINGS

Most chest freezers have a dial or knob featured as a "temperature control." These dials are not connected to a thermostat and do give helpful information about the actual temperature inside.

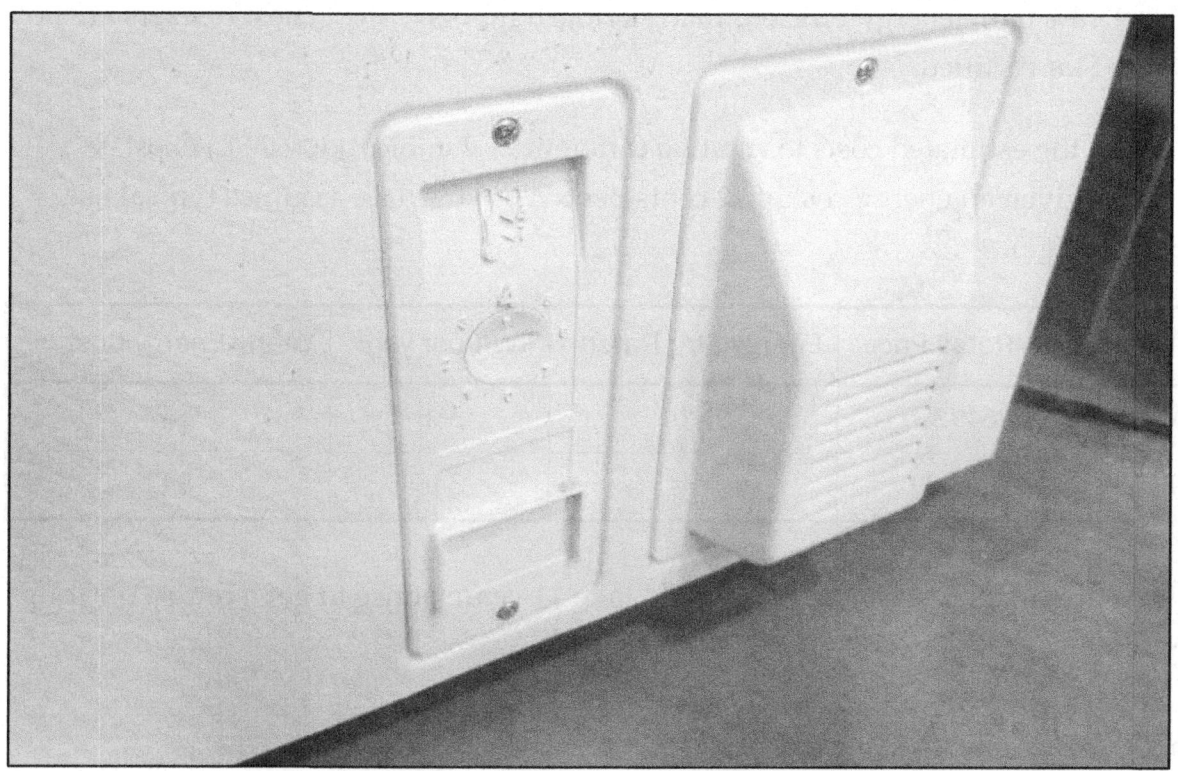

Whirlpool chest freezer controller dial

Some have simple options labelled "Minimum – Off – Maximum." Others are not as clear. For example, one chest freezer dial had the number "1 – 7." Which one is colder, "1" or "7"?

You need to read the manual to find out.

After your freezer is set up, place the dial on the coldest setting and leave it there. The reason for doing this is that having it on the coldest setting chills your water in the least amount of time, which means less wear on the compressor.

8. ENERGY EFFICIENCY RATINGS

I believe it is essential to be "green" and to consider our environment. That said, the upfront expense of "green" products can make them cost-prohibitive.

In the US, products can receive an "Energy Star" rating, which means that they are at least 10% more energy-efficient than standard models. Most chest freezers are not Energy Star certified.

Here are the estimated costs to run two different 21.7 cubic foot (600 L) chest freezers, given an energy cost of 12 cents per kWh. This data assumes typical use (food storage).

Brand	Retail Price	Energy Star Rated	kWh per year	Yearly Energy Cost
Whirlpool	$649.99	No	386	$47
GE	$854.99	Yes	346	$42

With a price difference of $205, it would take 41 years of use to get a return on your investment.

The final decision, of course, is yours to make.

Real World Setup

Ian is a chiropractor and martial artist and in the USA. He posted the following:

"THINGS LEARNED IN 2019 ABOUT CHEST FREEZER COLD WATER IMMERSION

1. Always unplug the freezer before getting in.

2. Sand the seams before using JB water weld to seal the inside of the freezer.

3. Always tighten the inner plug or even JB weld it shut to avoid external leaks.

4. The best way to avoid ice build-up is using an aquarium filter to cycle the water and set the freezer setting to cold versus coldest.

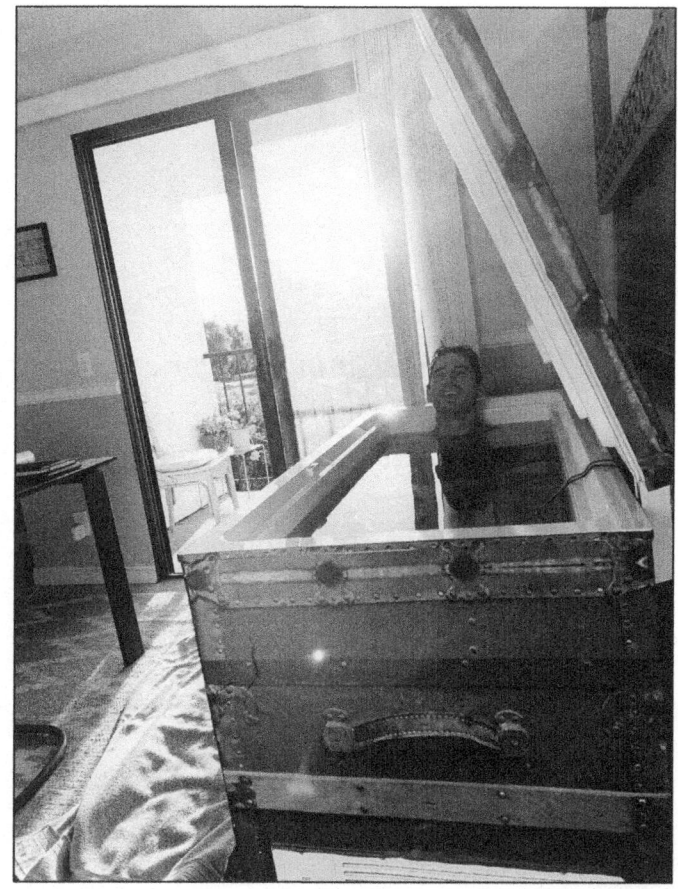

Ian Rassel

5. The best way to warm your body after an immersion is 30 seconds to 3 minutes of horse stance.

6. Utilizing breath techniques like Wim Hof or Pranayama is an excellent way of managing the cold.

7. Using fresh water with thirty or so drops of eucalyptus oil is amazing! Using 50 pounds of Epsom salt is great on the joints and skin but inconvenient to wash off and maintain.

8. Putting a wrap on the outside of the chest freezer is super challenging and definitely worth it. Highly recommend Randy at RM wraps.

9. John Richter is the oracle of chest freezer cold plunge questions. Thanks for the awesome manual John!!

10. Leave your timer alone after you get the hang of it. The ego always gets us into trouble and is not necessary in the cold. Whether it's one minute or ten it doesn't matter just get in."

" To get anywhere, or even to live a long time, *"*

a man has to guess, and guess right, over and over again,

without enough data for a logical answer.

Robert Heinlein

Chapter 4: Waterproofing - Seal the Seams

◼ THE IMPORTANCE OF SEALING THE SEAMS

"An ounce of prevention is worth a pound of cure."

Benjamin Franklin

I'm still surprised by the number of people who buy a chest freezer, make no changes, fill it with water, and gleefully report that it "works great."

A few are critical or dismissive about those who take time and money to seal their freezer or install liners. I have yet to see a single follow-up comment that their chest freezer still "works great" (or at all) a year later.

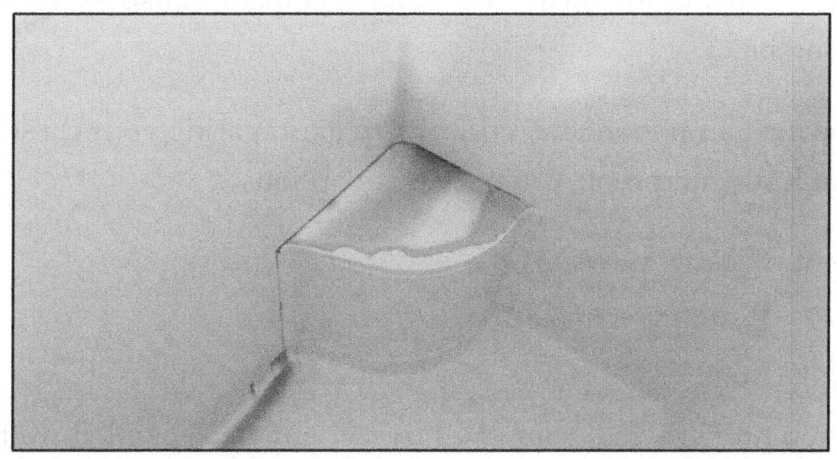

Rust!

As mentioned before, chest freezers are not designed to hold water. To protect your investment of time and money, you need to prepare your chest freezer to hold water.

If you don't seal the seams inside the chest freezer, water will seep into the inside walls. You may or may not see rust leaking from your seams immediately. However, over time, water will find its way inside.

Moisture rusts the inside walls or structure, erodes the insulation, damages the refrigeration coils, and causes the chest freezer to break down.

One common issue discussed on other forums about chest freezers (keezers, bait freezers, and regular food storage) is dealing with oxidation, or rust. If your chest freezer lasts long enough, rust is likely to happen. Why?

Moisture from the frost that builds up eventually gets inside the walls. Also, every time the lid opens, warmer air from outside mixes with the cold air inside, creating condensation.

If chest freezers used for their *intended* purpose end up with rust problems, you can be sure that filling them with water is going to cause issues… unless you take action beforehand.

The most important and critical step in preparing your chest freezer is to make sure that it is waterproof. You have three options:

1. Sealing the seams,
2. Installing a liner, or
3. Both.

If you properly seal your chest freezer and have painted walls, a liner is not completely necessary. However, installing a liner does add another layer of protection, and will likely increase the life of your chest freezer. If you have unpainted (bare metal) walls, a liner is a strongly recommended.

If you choose to install a liner, I still recommend that you seal the seams. Why? If the liner ever gets punctured or cracks, or water splashes into your chest freezer while you are removing your liner for cleaning, water can get into the seams. If your seams are sealed, that will not be an issue. Sealing your seams also prevents condensation from getting inside the walls.

Chest freezers have a number of seams in different places, depending on the brand and model. Most new chest freezers have seams where the floor meets the bottom of the wall and around the compressor cover. There are typically one or two vertical seams (bottom to top) where the wall sections meet.

Find the seams by looking and feeling for two pieces of metal coming together. Sometimes one piece of metal is bent or curved around a corner. Other times it can be two pieces that overlap.

The seams may fit tightly together, or there may be a gap. If the gap of any seam is larger than 1/4-inch (6.3 mm), it may be difficult or impossible to get your sealant to fill that much space. It is best to return the chest freezer and get one with smaller (or no) gaps.

The following pictures show seams from a few chest freezers.

The 15-cu. ft. Whirlpool chest freezer has seams where all walls meet the floor, one vertical seam from bottom to top on the front wall, and seams around the cover over the compressor. The corners of the walls are curved and do not have seams.

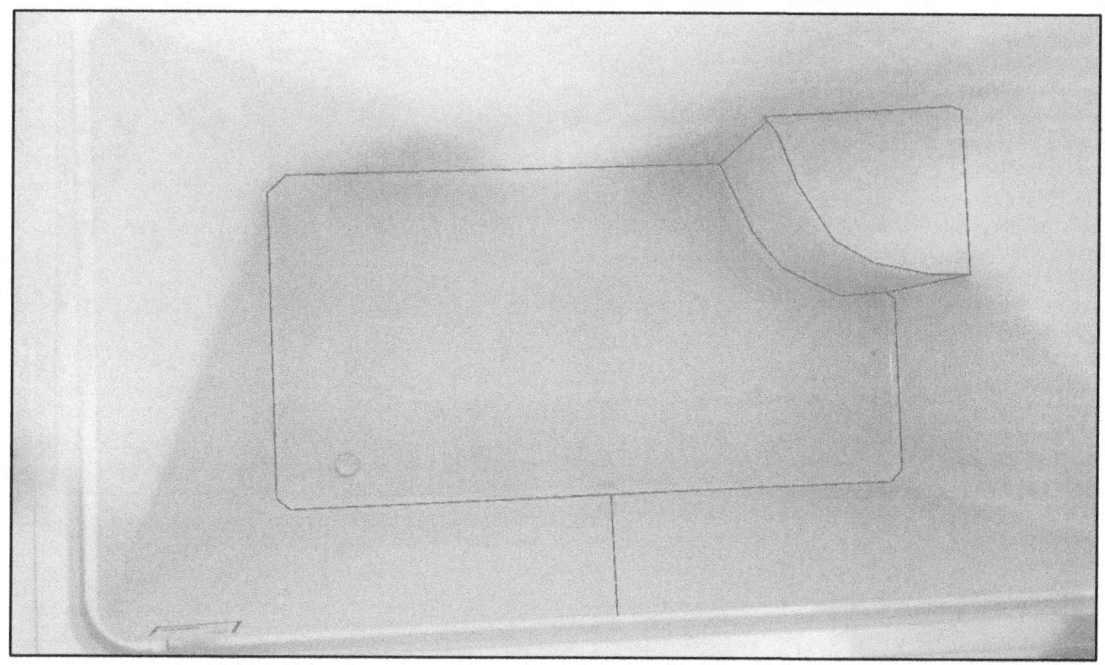

Whirlpool seams marked in red

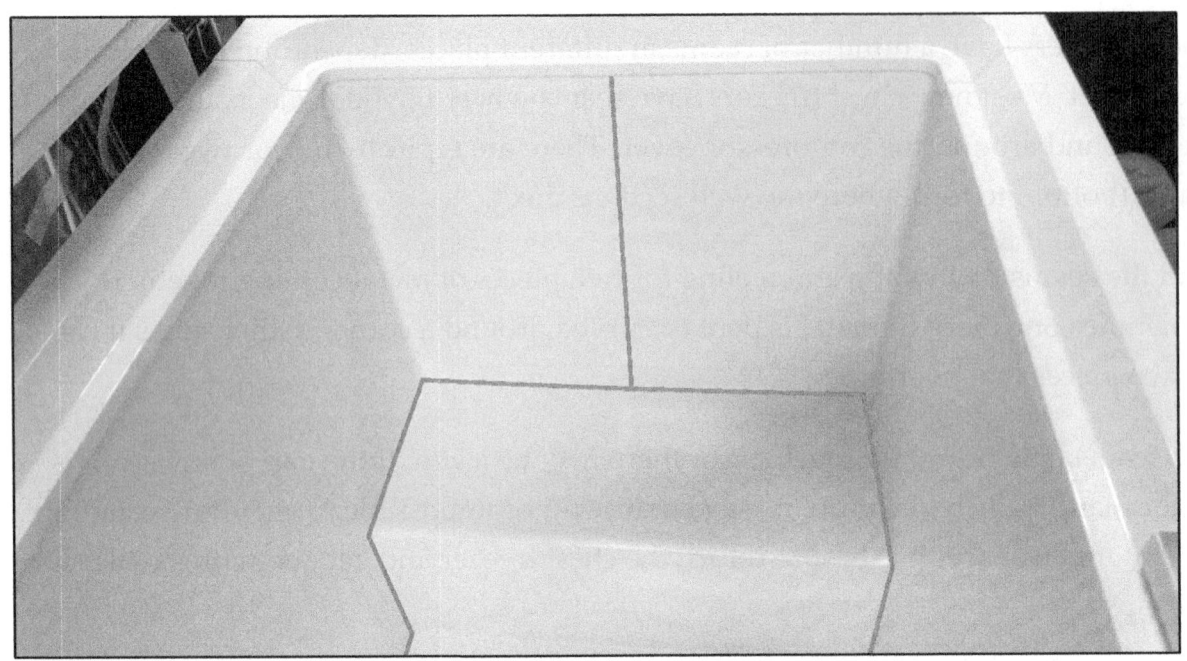

Frigidaire seams around the compressor

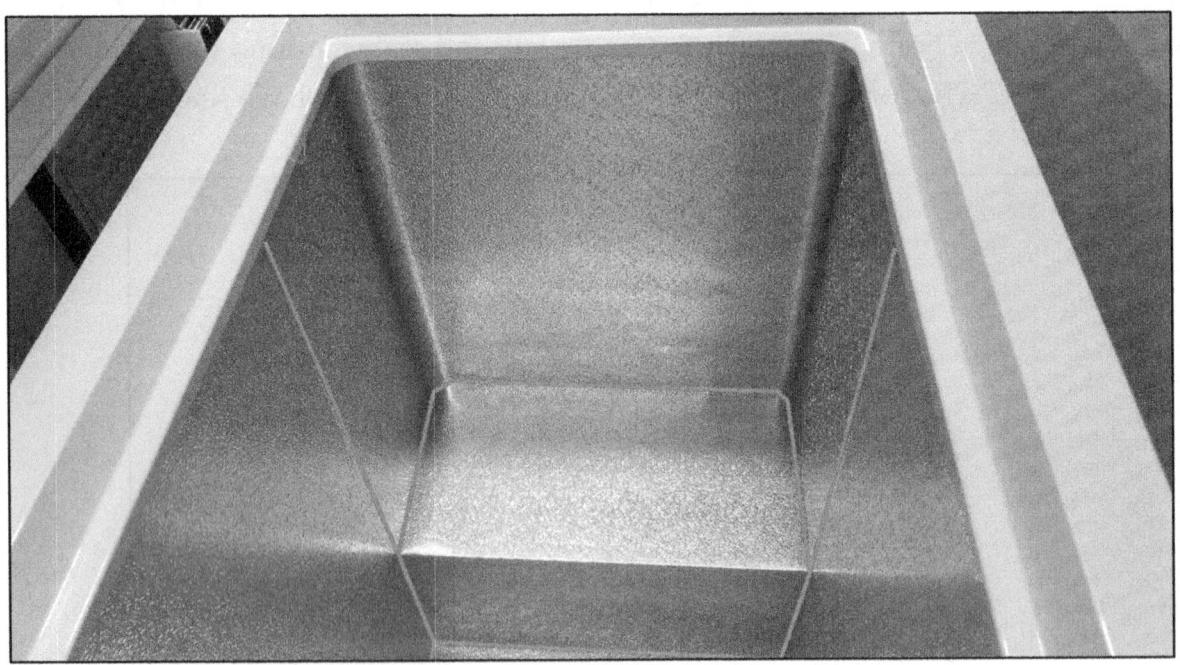

Seams on an unpainted freezer

The walls and floor seams on the Whirlpool models overlap.

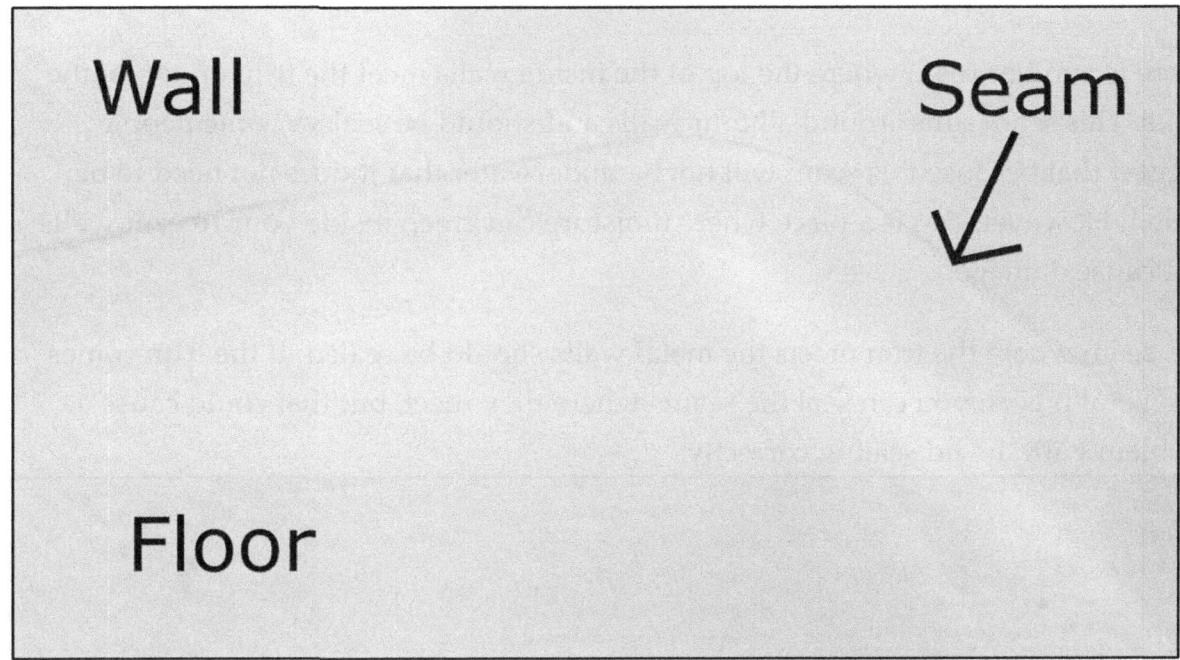

Floor and wall seams - Whirlpool

The wall and floor seams on Frigidaire models abut.

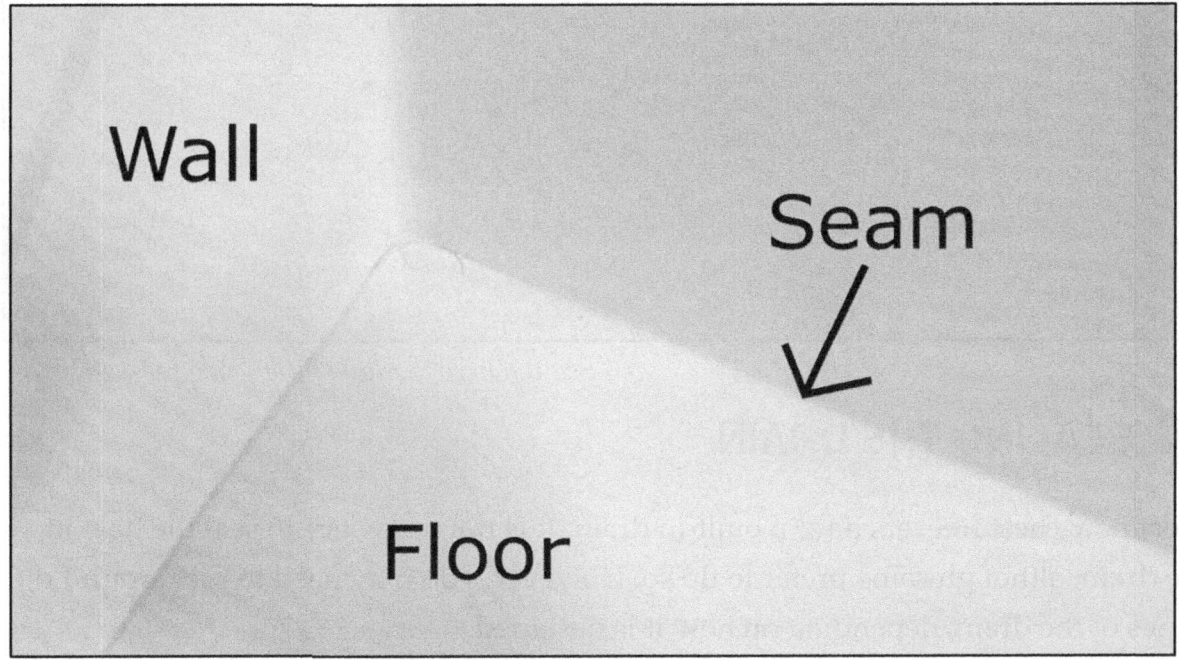

Floor and walls - Frigidaire

THE UPPER WALL SEAM

There is another seam where the top of the inside walls meet the trim on top of the walls. This seam runs around all four walls and should be sealed. Some people suggest that because this seam will not be underwater that it does not need to be sealed. However, this is a place where moisture can creep inside your freezer walls and cause damage.

The seam where the trim meets the metal walls should be sealed. If the trim comes in several pieces, you can seal the seams where they meet, but that could cause a problem with the lid sealing correctly.

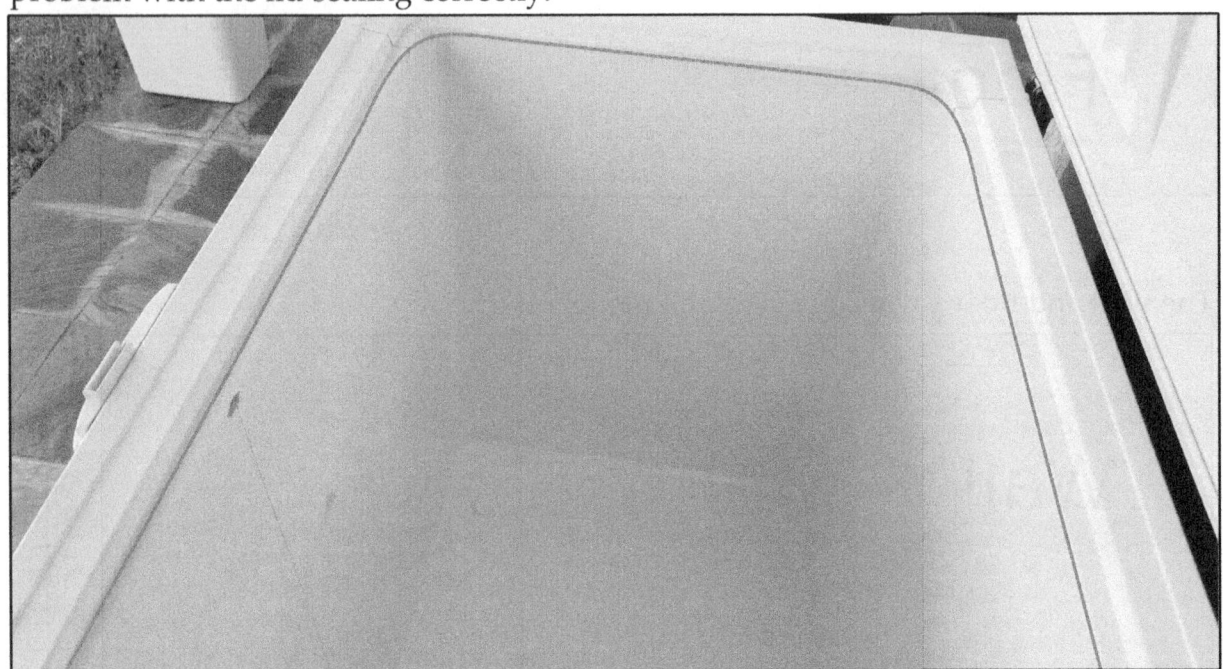

Seam where the top of the walls meet the trim

 ## SEALING THE DRAIN

Most new chest freezers have a built-in drain. It is not necessary to seal the hole in the drain, although some prefer to do so. However, you may need to seal around the edges of the drain, depending on how it is designed.

On some freezers, the outer edge surrounding the drain is built into the same piece of material as the floor, has no seams, and does not need to be sealed.

On other freezers, the area around the drain is a separate piece of metal and should be sealed. Refer to the below diagrams and look at your chest freezer closely to see what needs to be done.

Chest freezers have two drain plugs, one inside on the floor, and one outside on the front wall. Some drains work better than others at keeping water in your chest freezer.

If water leaks from your drain, there are two possible causes. The seam around the drain plug is not sealed, or the plug is not fitting snugly enough.

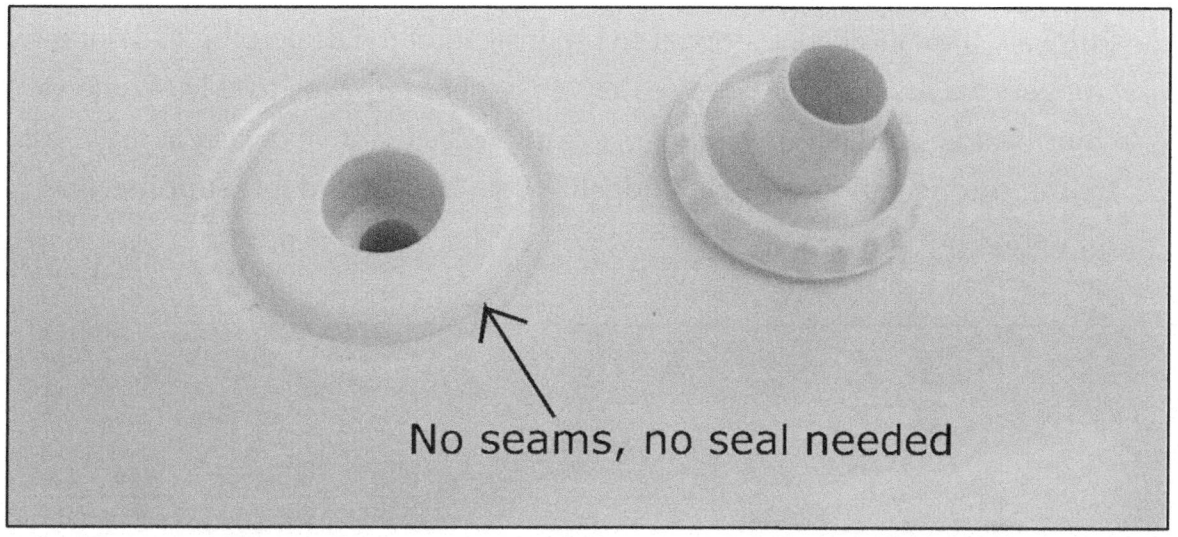

No seams, no seal needed

Seamless drain

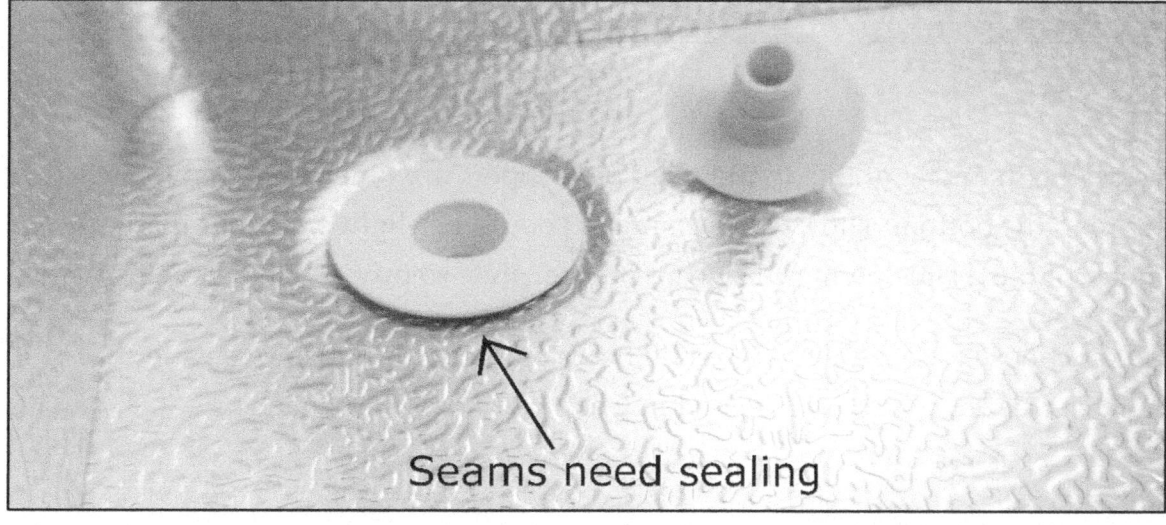

Seams need sealing

Frigidaire Drain with seams

If there is a seam around the plug opening, seal it along with the other seams, but leave enough room for the drain plug to still be removed and replaced.

If that does not solve the problem, then the drain plug is not closing tightly enough. There are two fixes:

1. Take the inside drain plug to your local hardware or plumbing store and find a thin silicone gasket that will fit around the stem of the plug. Do not buy a gasket made of rubber because it can crack in the cold and is not compatible with ozone.

2. Purchase a small silicone stopper to use instead of the drain plug. Do not buy stoppers made of rubber because they do not hold up well to cold, ozone, or chlorine. I've used several stoppers to plug holes that I've drilled in my chest freezer during various setups. WidgetCo.com is an affordable supplier, and they ship quickly.

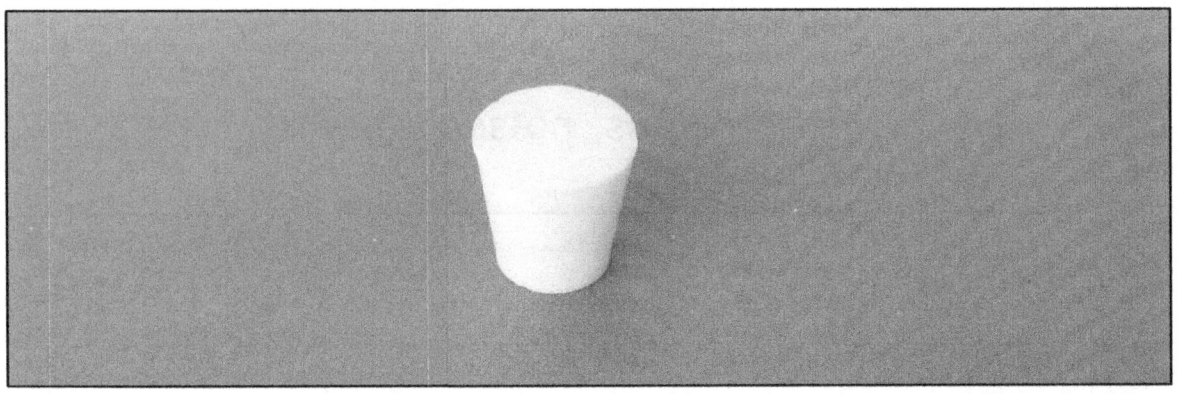

Silicon stopper

Measure the diameter of the drain hole. The stoppers are tapered so that the top is wider than the bottom. The bottom diameter should be slightly smaller than the diameter of the drain opening. They are inexpensive, so buy a few to have on hand.

If you do choose to seal the drain, you'll need another way to remove water from your chest freezer, which is discussed in Chapter 15 on Maintenance.

◼ AVAILABLE PRODUCTS

There are dozens of sealants and adhesives available. Most are not suitable for a cold plunge application. This section will discuss common options and how to prepare the surface for sealing.

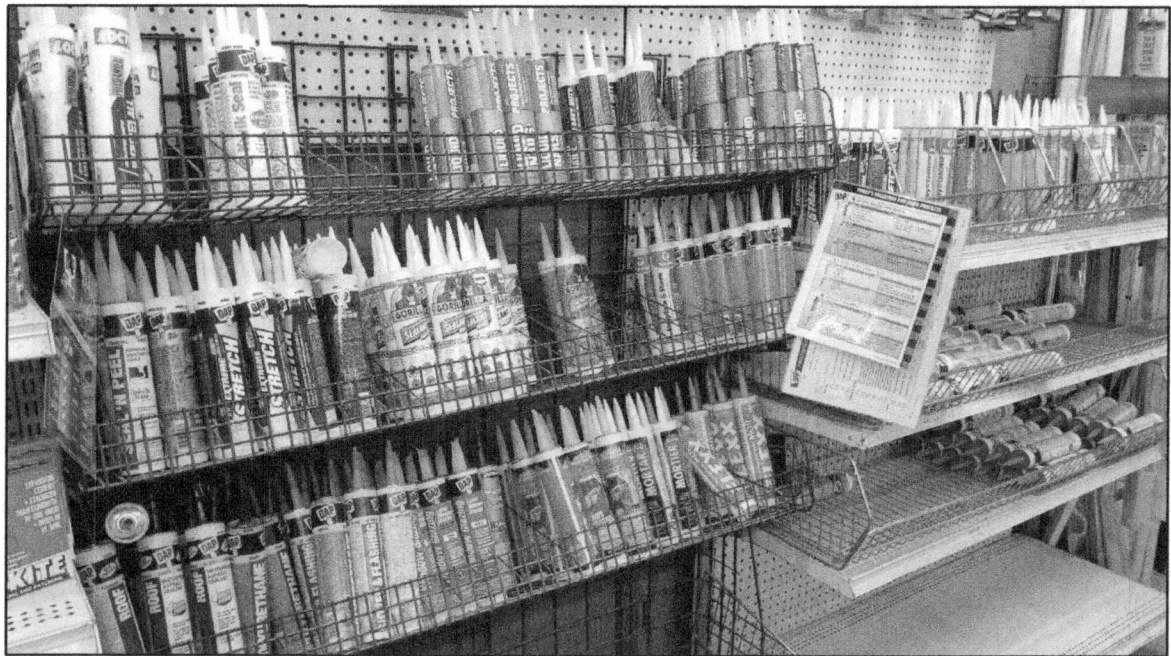

A wall of sealants to avoid

◼ Preparing the Surface

Before applying any sealant, clean the inside of your chest freezer. Use dish detergent and a soft sponge. Stronger products are not necessary.

Read the directions on the sealant tube or package to find out if other steps are needed.

Correctly preparing the surface before applying any sealant is a critical step. The three most common reasons for sealants to fail are:

1. Using the wrong product,
2. Not correctly preparing the surface, and
3. Poor workmanship.

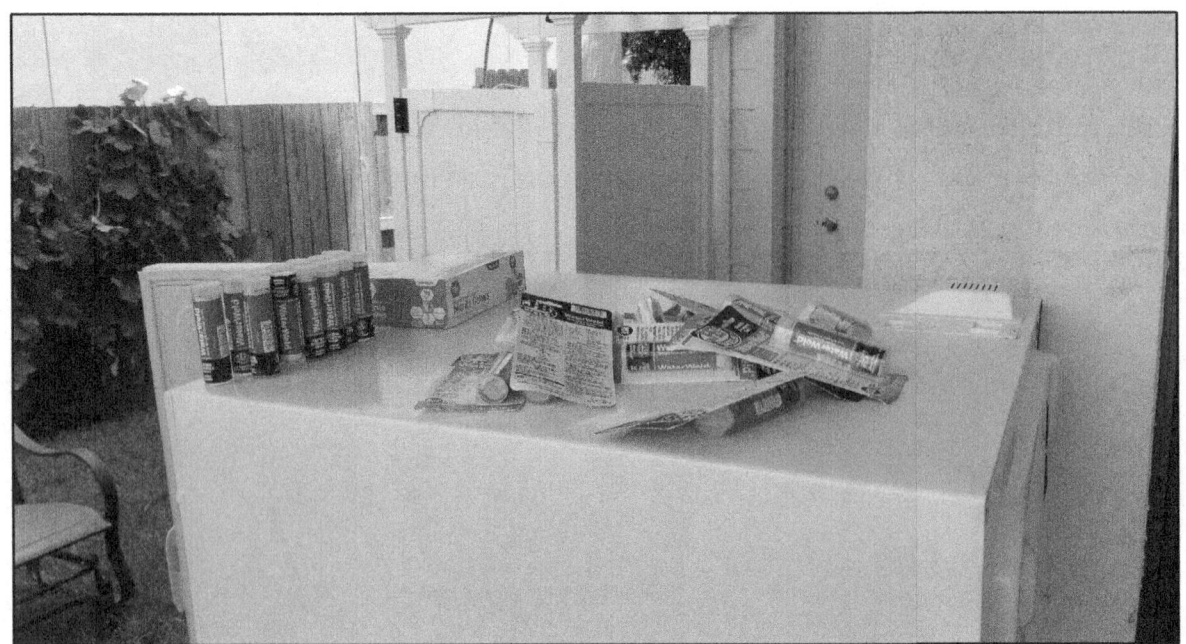

Getting ready to seal with JB Water Weld

■ JB Water Weld

JB water Weld (JBWW) is my top recommendation for sealing. I have yet to have a negative report about JBWW when it has been correctly applied.

It is a two-part epoxy that comes in a stick of putty. If you are in part of the world where JBWW is not available, look for a product called "Selleys Knead it Aqua." It seems to be comparable.

JBWW sets in about 15-25 minutes, so work in small quantities. It cures within 1 hour and dries hard. However, to be on the safe side, I recommend letting it sit for 24 hours before you add water. After it dries, it is non-toxic, has a tensile strength of 900 psi, and is reported to be stronger than steel.

If you prepare the surface correctly, and the putty is mixed and applied correctly, it will most likely last longer than your chest freezer.

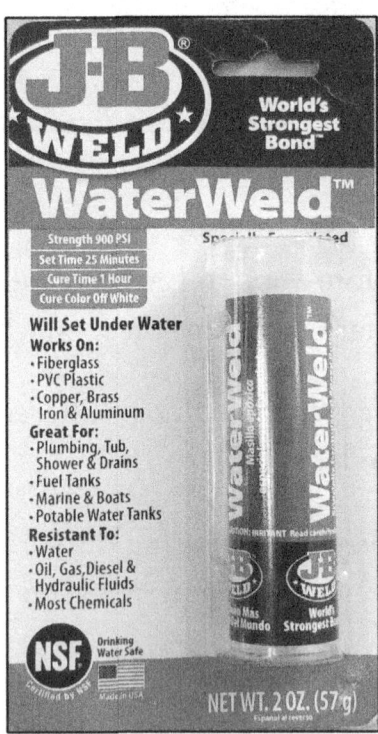

Use JB Water Weld

There are no contraindications that I know of for using JBWW. It has no odor after drying. It is not affected by salts, hydrogen peroxide, ozone, or UV light. After it cures, no chemicals leach into the water, and it is safe for people who have chemical sensitivities.

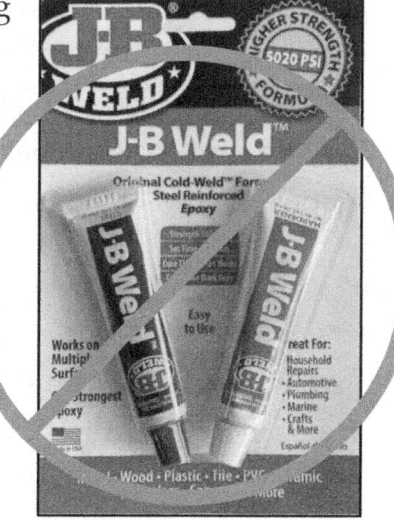

Do NOT Use the Basic JB Weld Product

How Many Tubes Does It Take?

Depending upon the size of your chest freezer and how liberally you apply it, you might need between 15 to 25 tubes. Sealing the seams around the top wall of the chest freezer is recommended, even if they are not underwater. If you want to seal these seams with JBWW, it might take an additional six to eight tubes. Measure all of your seams to figure out how many tubes are needed.

The line of putty over the seams should be about 1" (2.5 cm) wide, and about 1/8" (.3 cm) thick. One tube of JB Water weld covers about 16 inches (40.6 cm) of seams.

Using those guidelines, one tube of JBWW covers approximately 16 inches (40 cm) of seams. A 15 cubic foot (400 L) Whirlpool chest freezer, has about 230 inches (584 cm) of seams. 15 – 18 tubes will seal all of the seams on the walls, the floor, and around the compressor cabinet. Sealing the seams between the top edge of the wall and the top molding will take about 10-12 tubes.

Since these seams are not submerged, if you want to save a few dollars you can use silicone. See the section later in this chapter for more information.

Prepping Your Chest Freezer for Work

Turning the chest freezer on its side makes it easier to crawl into for working. Put down a blanket and get another person to help you gently move it into place. Be sure to place it on the side that is a solid piece of metal- not the side with the temperature control of vents.

Besides cleaning your chest freezer, JBWW recommends that you lightly sand the area where it will be applied. Use finishing sandpaper – 120 grit should be fine. The manufacturer recommends to sand off the paint entirely on either side of the seam. However, reports so far indicate that this is not necessary. If you have a chest freezer with a painted interior, lightly sand enough to rough up the paint a bit.

Where two walls come together at a 90-degree angle, I found it easier to cut the sandpaper into a small rectangle, about 2" x 4" (5 – 10 cm) and roll it into a tube. This way you can lightly sand both walls at the same time moving the sandpaper tube parallel to the seam.

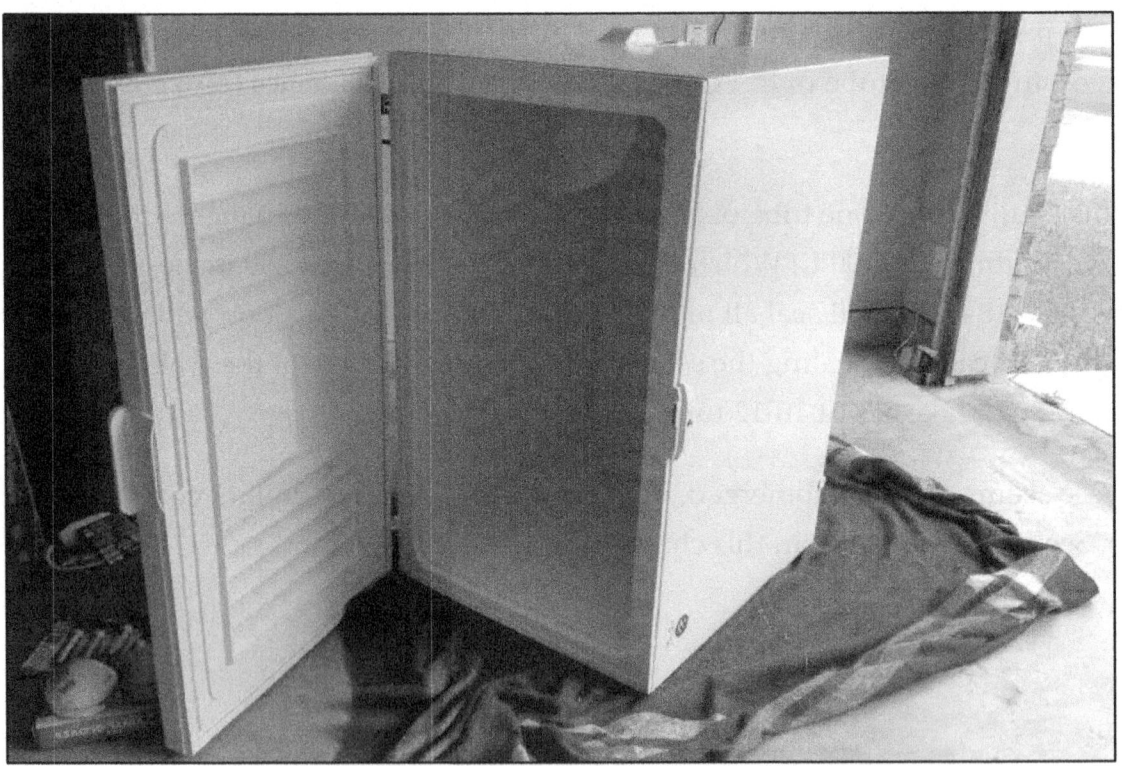

Ready for work!

After sanding, sweep or vacuum the residue and wipe the seams with a mild cleaner. While it is not necessary for the surface to dry before applying the putty, it makes me feel better to wait.

What to Do If You Accidentally Sand Off the Paint

If you accidentally sand through the paint and see bare metal underneath, that is okay. Cover any exposed metal with JBWW. If you notice any scratches in the paint that expose the metal underneath, apply JBWW.

Getting Ready to Apply

I prefer to wear gloves when working with sealants because I don't like them to get it on my skin. As you work, the residue cures on the gloves, making it challenging to mix new putty. Buy a box of 100 disposable gloves for the project. Vinyl or nitrile are best. Latex can work but are more likely to tear and tend to gunk up with putty sooner. Latex gloves are pictured below. You might also use thicker mechanics gloves because they are easier to work with. Get gloves that are smooth, not textured.

> ## TIPS
>
> 1. Wearing several layers of gloves can speed up your workflow. As the putty hardens, remove the outside layer.
>
> Gloves with powder on the inside are *much* easier to put on!
>
> 2. You can put water on the gloves to reduce the amount of putty that sticks to the gloves. Do NOT use soap or any other chemical- only water.

It is OK to dampen your gloves with plain water. Do *not* use acetone, lacquer thinner, mineral spirits, soap or any other type of fluid because it could prevent the product from curing.

If you do not wear gloves, wash the JBWW from your fingers, and clean underneath your fingernails before it cures. Do not wait any longer than 15 minutes. After it cures, it is much harder to remove. That is another reason why I prefer to wear gloves – they are fast to remove and replace and keep your workflow going.

Before it cures, the putty emits a slight odor, which can build up inside the chest freezer. Work in a well-ventilated space. If you are sensitive to chemical smells, consider setting up an oscillating fan.

Mixing the Putty

The putty has two parts. The outer part is a whitish color, and the inner part is gray. Work in small quantities.

While it is not necessary to have a very thick application of JBWW for it to work, it will not hurt anything if you use too much. However, it is important not to spread the putty too thinly.

> **TIP**
>
> Thoroughly mix the putty! Do not be in a hurry. It is always easier to do it right the first time than to have to do it a second time.

To apply the putty, pinch off about half an inch (13 mm) from the stick. Thoroughly mix it by flattening it and folding it over several times. It is wholly mixed when the color is uniform. If you see any streaks of gray, the putty is not mixed enough and will not cure. Keep mixing!

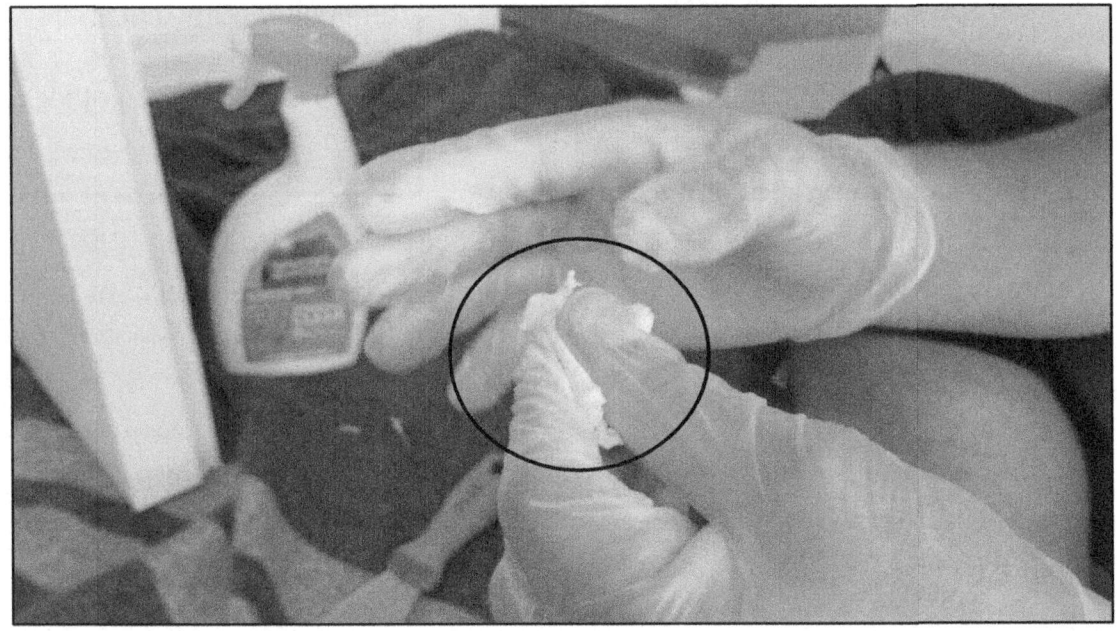

Mixing Water Weld

Once the putty is thoroughly mixed, roll it into a ball and then roll the ball between your hands to form a snake-like shape. You probably did this as a kid with Play-Doh. Make a putty snake between 3 – 5 inches (7 – 13 cm) long and close to 1/4" (~6 mm) thick.

Applying the Putty

Take your putty snake and push it into the seam. Spread it about 1/2" (12.7 mm) on each side of the seam. A little more or less than that is fine. Again, it is better to apply too much than too little.

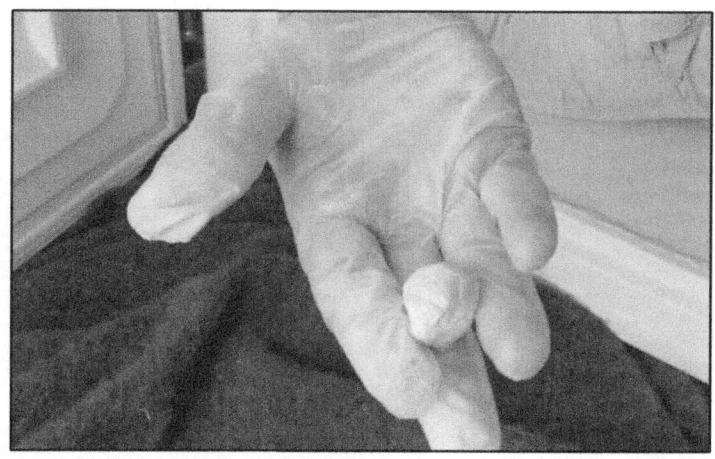

Putty ball

Place the putty snake along the seam. Spread it one direction along the seam, left or right. Be sure that there are no bubbles or gaps along the edges where the putty meets the walls.

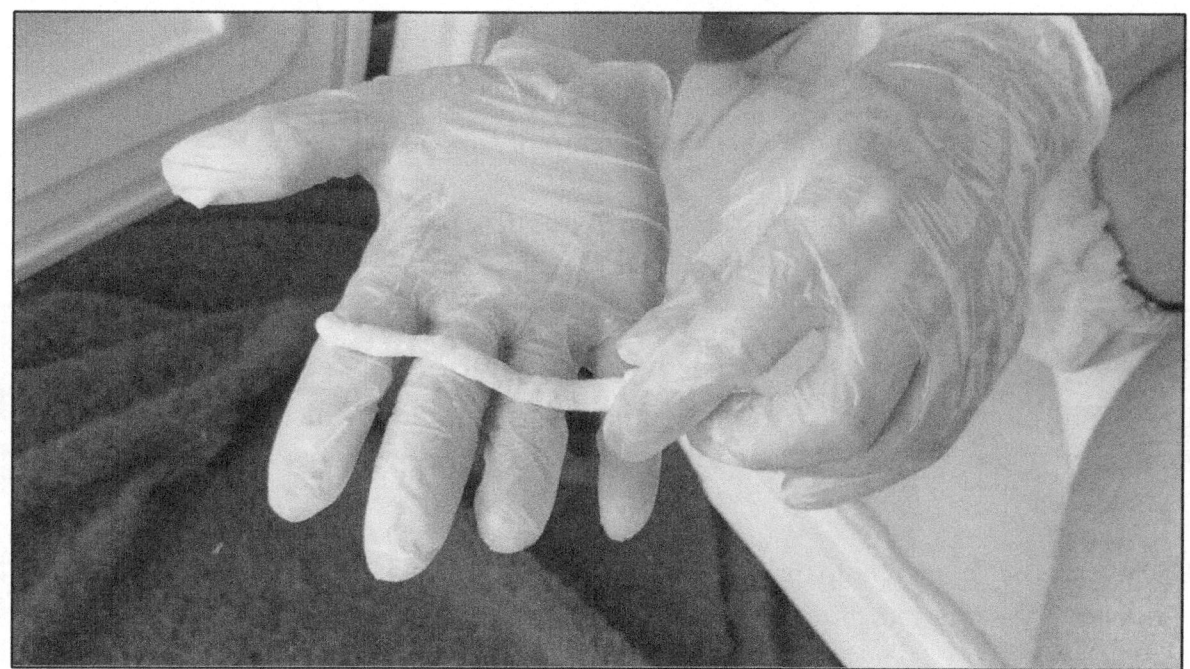

Putty snake

Work in one direction until you reach the end of the seam or back to where you started.

Be sure that each new bit of putty snake overlaps the previously applied putty to ensure a proper seal.

Using one finger in a rolling motion, roll one edge of the JB weld away from the seam, so that it spreads away from the seam. Ensure that there are no gaps. Do the same thing on the opposite side.

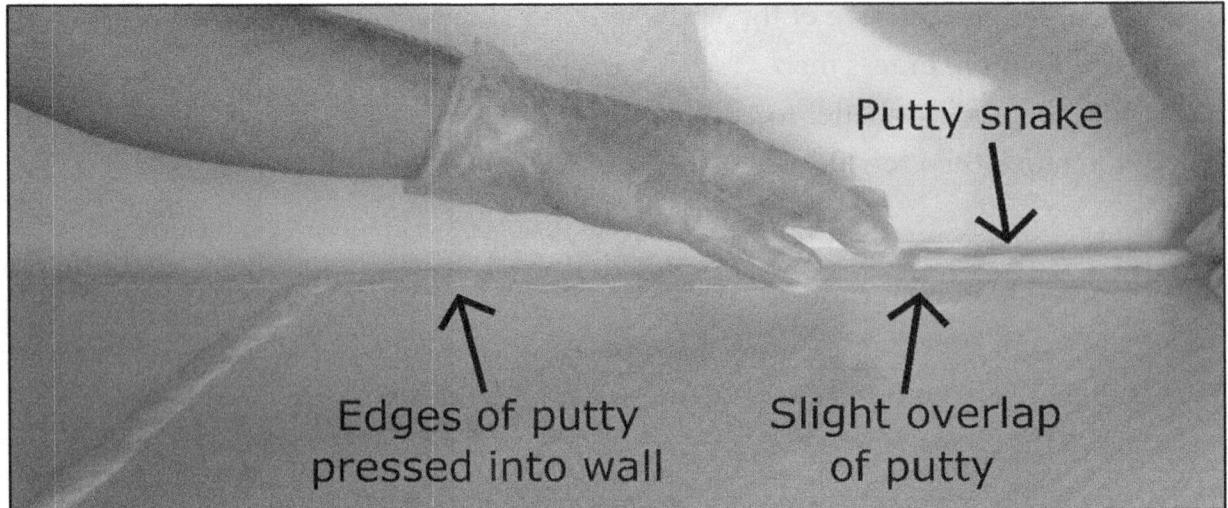

Applying the putty snake

Repeat this process until you seal all of the seams.

There are videos posted on the Facebook group of this process.

After you finish, let the chest freezer sit with the lid open for 24 hours.

HOW LONG DOES IT TAKE?

Depending on the length of seams in your chest freezer, how focused you are, and a number of other variables, it could take anywhere from 5 – 8 hours to seal all of the seams.

Having another person help mix the putty will move things along much faster. However, don't let them get ahead of you- once the JB Water Weld starts to cure it will not stick

Double Check Your Work

After 24 hours, visually and physically inspect the JBWW. All of the putty should be hard to the touch with no sponginess. It should also be a consistent off-white color. If it is the slightest bit soft or has any gray streaks in it, this means that it was not mixed properly and needs to be removed.

What to Do if the JB Water Weld Did Not Cure Properly

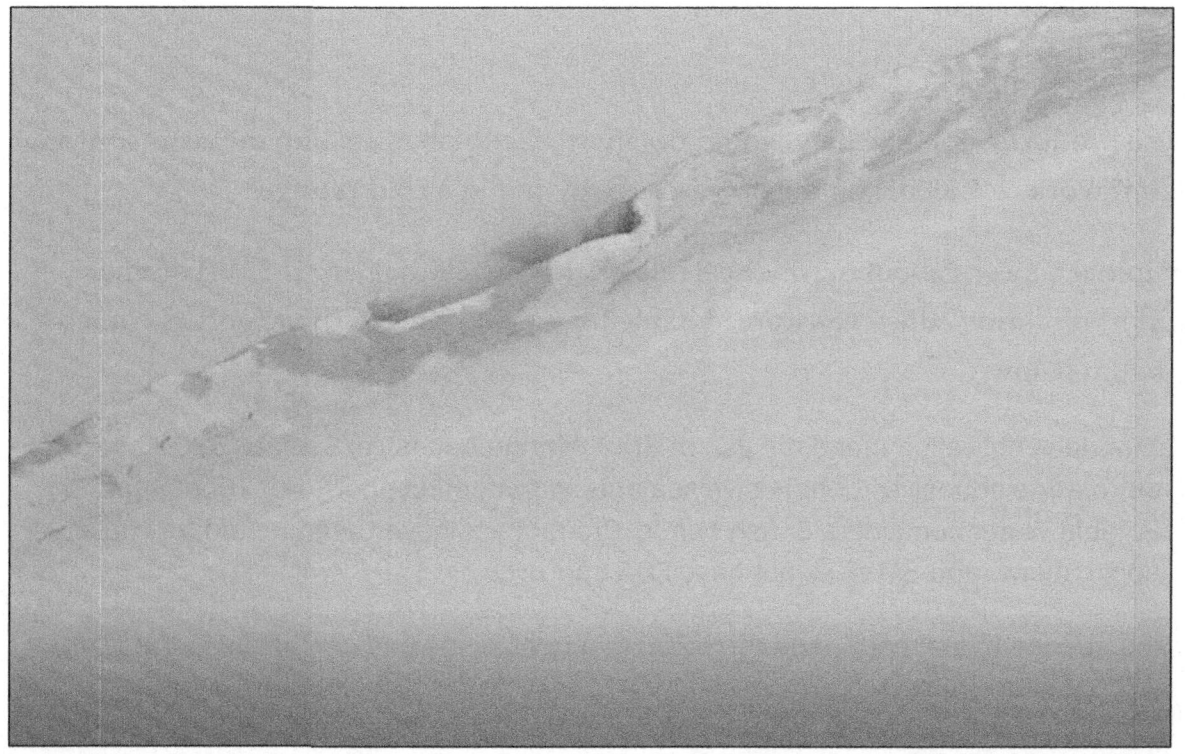

Grey streaks = unmixed putty

Removing JBWW is not easy or fun and brings a risk of scraping off your paint and denting your chest freezer's walls or floors.

If you have to remove any uncured JBWW, use a small putty knife, carefully scraping toward the seam. Then sand the area again and clean with a degreaser or denatured alcohol to remove all of the uncured putty.

Throw away the putty that did not cure – it cannot be reused. Reapply new putty to the areas needed. Overlap the new putty with JBWW that has already cured.

Price & Alternative Products

In the US, one tube of JBWW costs between $4 - $7 per tube, which means your entire cost to seal all inside seams should be less than or close to $100 for a 15-cu. ft. (424 L) freezer.

In countries outside of the US, JBWW can cost as much as $18 - $21 per tube. Our friends in Australia have used "Selleys Knead It Aqua" product, and so far, it seems to be working great.

■ Marine Adhesive Sealants

These products look like they would do an excellent job of sealing the seams. After all, if it works for a boat on the open seas, why not in a cold plunge?

My initial concern about marine sealants relates to health. I asked 3M customer support if marine adhesives were suitable for a cold plunge. Their reply is copied verbatim below:

> "3M does not recommend the use of 3M™ Marine Adhesive/Sealant 5200 or any of our marine adhesives or adhesive sealants in swimming pools, Hot Tubs, Spas, or Potable Water containers or fish ponds. Product has never been tested for these applications, and 3M does not have FDA approval.

> If someone has already used the 5200 in a pool, acids and chemicals in the water will break down the sealant causing particles to float which could be ingested."

Bottom line: do *NOT* use these products. More information is on the MSDS, including the chemicals that are probable and known carcinogens- in particular, isocyanates.

■ 100% silicone

Many people have used silicone to seal their chest freezer. It has the advantage of being readily available, simple to apply, and inexpensive. Many fish enthusiasts use 100% pure silicone labeled for aquarium use. I have had one report from a member in our group of a silicone-sealed chest freezer with reported leaks for two years.

However, there are a number of potential problems to be aware of, and silicone products in *general* have the largest number of reported failures from members of our Facebook group.

There are many different types and grades of silicone products. Typically, anything sold at a big-box or local hardware stores is not going to produce good results.

Besides not using a high-quality silicone product meant for long-term underwater use, there are a few other reasons that could cause silicone to fail:

1. Not correctly preparing the work surface
2. Insufficient cleaning of the work surface before applying
3. Incorrectly applying the silicone (too thin or thick, or unevenly)
4. Not letting is cure long enough before adding water.
5. Using chlorine or other chemicals that deteriorate silicone

Because of these reasons, I do not recommend silicone for new chest freezers unless you are experienced and know what you are doing. I am including information here primarily for those who want an inexpensive way to seal used chest freezers that will also use a pond liner or other type of liner.

Currently, two members of our group have reported good short-term results from a commercial grade product called Sikasil-Pool, which is used to seal swimming pools. I am cautiously optimistic, and will update the book and Facebook group after we have long-term (12+ months) reports of success.

Types of Silicone

There are many posts on aquarium forums about the difference between "regular" 100% silicone and that labeled for aquarium use. Most say there is no difference. Some fish owners have alleged that this is a marketing gimmick to double or triple the price. However, there may be a difference in how it cures, which could be critical.

I honestly do not know if there is any difference.

If you are sensitive to chemicals, avoid silicone that mentions any of the following on the label:

- Mold resistant,

- Mold-free,

- Fungicide,

- Bacteria protection,

- Anti-microbial

Read the label carefully, because even if it says "100% Pure Silicone" it may contain toxic additives.

Pros and Cons of Using Silicone

While epoxy putties like JB Water Weld have the largest number of reported successes for sealing chest freezers, silicone does have many advocates, although I am still hesitant to recommend it for the reasons already mentioned. When it comes to any construction project that you plan to keep or use for the long term, I believe it is always best (and far less expensive) to do things right the first time than fix mistakes and start over. For that reason, I recommend epoxy putty first.

JB water Weld costs only $50 - $100 more than silicone. I know it is more expensive outside of the US. While it does take longer to apply, if you intend to have your chest freezer for a long time, in my opinion, it is worth it.

If the gap in the seam is more than 1/4 in. (6 mm) wide or deep, silicone is not recommended, and JB Water Weld should be used instead.

Some of the reasons I don't recommend silicone include:

1. A lifetime of noticing showers and bathtubs where the silicone caulking needs to be replaced every few years.

2. Several manufacturers state they do not recommend silicone for prolonged water immersion.

3. Some manufacturers stated that their silicone was only okay if used in tanks with less than 30 gallons (114 L).

4. A growing number of people in our Facebook group are reporting rust leaking from their chest freezer a few months after sealing with silicone. This problem could be attributed to insufficient preparation of the surface, poor application, or the silicone itself, or reactions with chemicals or devices used for sanitation.

> **CAUTION**
>
> Do not seal your freezer with silicone if you plan to use chlorine for water sanitation because there is poor compatibility.

Checking with the Manufacturers

I sent emails to four manufacturers of silicone products, GE, DAP, 3M, and Momentive. I heard back from all but GE. I asked them if they could recommend a product for a custom home-made cold plunge that met the following requirements:

- Aluminum or painted steel walls

- Volume: 100 - 200 gallons (379 - 757 L)

- Water temperature: 30 - 40° F (-1.1 - 4.4° C)

- Safety Requirements: Must not leach any chemicals in the water.

- Water-proof: Must work for prolonged submersion

- Must hold up well with various water sanitation methods including chlorine, bromine, ozone, UV-C light, and salts.

3M and DAP replied that their products are not suitable or recommended.

The engineer from Momentive said that their RTV100 series "...may work for your application." Did you notice the hedge words: "may work..."? They did not say it would be perfect or even provide a simple "yes" answer. This gives me a little cause for concern, but maybe I'm being overcautious, and they are just avoiding liability.

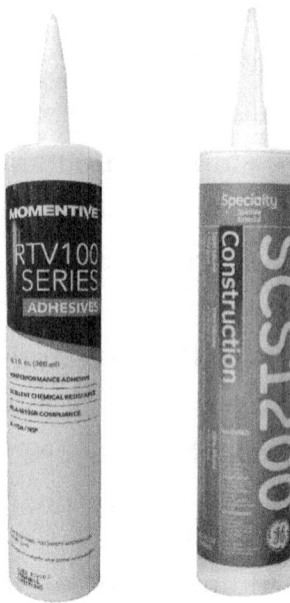

If you still insist on using silicone, people who build fish tanks recommend two types:

1. Momentive RTV100 series

2. GE 1200 Series Construction Sealant

The Momentive product is food safe. It will release gas chemicals before curing, but not afterward.

Tubes of silicon

Purchase the Momentive RTV100 series from specialty stores or online. It comes in four colors.

Product #/Color	Cartridge size	Price
RTV102 - White	10.3 oz. (305 ml)	$17 - $34
RTV103 - Black	10.1 oz. (299 ml)	$12 - $15
RTV108 - Translucent	10.1 oz. (299 ml)	$12 - $15
RTV109 - Silver	10.1 oz. (299 ml)	$12 - $15

When to Use Primer

Here is additional information from the Momentive engineer:

If you have an unpainted aluminum interior, using primer improves adhesion. Momentive has two that are recommended: SS4004 or SS4044. SS4004 has a pink color that makes it easier to see and apply evenly. If you don't want that discoloration, use the SS4044, which is clear. Without testing, it is unknown as to whether or not the adhesive would work on the painted interior with or without the primer. He suggested trying it first without the primer, but there are no guarantees.

These primers are sold in one-pint bottles at the cost of $84.

Be sure to check the manufacturer recommendations for other products. A primer might be required depending on the surface material of your chest freezer.

How Much to Use

The sealant must not be used in a thickness of greater than 1/4 in. (6 mm). One 10 oz. tube covers 20 - 24 feet (6 - 7 meters) with a 1/4 in. (6 mm) bead. One or two tubes will be enough to seal a chest freezer under 15-cu. ft. (424 L). Larger chest freezers require two or three tubes. If in doubt, it is better to have an extra tube than to run out.

Squeeze Tubes vs. Caulking Guns

Do not purchase the small squeezable tubes of silicone, but rather the larger tubes that require a caulking gun. The reason for this is to ensure a thick enough seal across the seam. Do your best to apply it evenly.

You can buy a cheap caulking gun for under $5, but I found them difficult to use. The triggers are hard to squeeze, the silicone tends to come out unevenly, too quickly, and drips afterward. Caulking guns priced at $15 - $20 are comfortable to squeeze, apply a consistent bead, and prevent dripping.

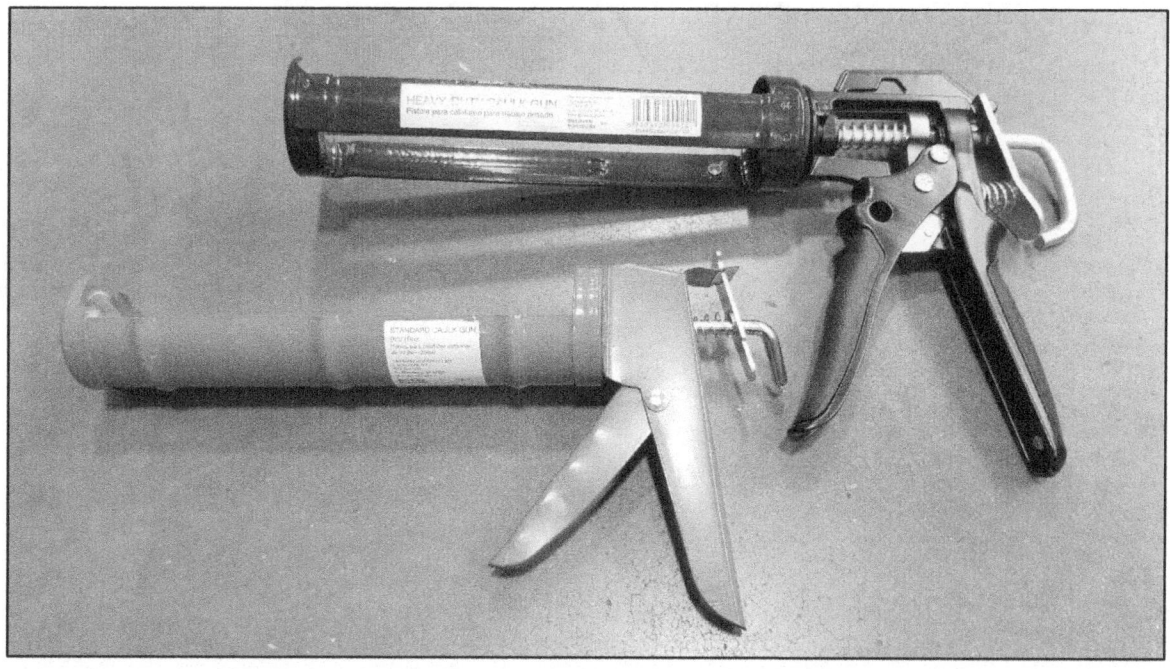

Cheap (bottom) and better (top) caulking guns

Applying Silicone

Applying silicone is relatively simple, but there are a number of things you need to keep in mind. Wearing latex or vinyl gloves prevents caulk from getting on your hands. It is not necessary to mask or put down tape, unless you just want straight lines.

1. Cut off the plastic end of the tube so that the hole is about 1/4 in. (6 mm) wide.

2. Use a nail or the tool on the caulking gun to break the seal inside of the plastic end that you just cut off.

3. Insert the tube into the caulking gun and press the plunger until it stops.

4. Hold the tip of the tube at a 45-degree angle to the seam, touching the seams to be sealed. It is best to pull the tube toward you. Pushing the tube away from you can result in an uneven application.

5. Squeeze the trigger slowly and move the gun toward you at a steady, even pace. When the trigger is pushed all the way in, release it. Repeat.

6. To stop the flow of caulk (when taking a break), pull the plunger away from the tube of caulk. Press it in before starting.

7. Apply it evenly over all of the seams and ensure that there are no gaps.

8. Do not run your finger across the silicone after you apply it because doing so thins the amount of silicone which weakens the seal. If you want to make it look neat, buy a "Caulking Tool" or make a caulking tool out of cardboard, or use a Popsicle stick. Run the edge of the tool along the bead of silicone to wipe away the excess and leave enough for a proper seal.

9. You have about 20 minutes until it is tack-free.

10. Quickly clean up spills with a rag and rubbing alcohol or mineral spirits. After it dries, excess silicone must be scraped off.

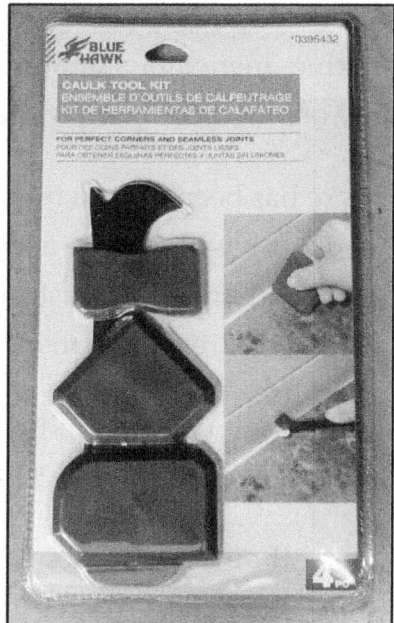

Caulking tool kit

11. The manufacturer says it takes three days to cure. Aquarium builders recommend letting it cure for seven days before you add water.

Keep in mind that unlike your shower, bathtub or kitchen, the seal on your chest freezer doesn't need to look pretty, and if you apply too much, that's OK. However, be careful, because too thick of an application may not cure properly. You can apply silicone to silicone that has not yet dried. New silicone applied to dried silicone will not seal correctly.

Apply only one bead of caulk. Adding more layers will not help.

When working with any chemical sealant, work in a well-ventilated area and wear gloves.

■ Epoxy Resin

There are countless epoxy products on the market. They can be used to coat art, furniture, floors, and boats, and other items. A few people have covered either the seams or the entire inside of their chest freezer with epoxy products.

Some key risks of using epoxy are that the process requires precise measuring, mixing, meticulous timing, special tools, and multiple layers to be done correctly. If any one of these many variables are off, your epoxy will fail.

There has been quite a bit of discussion with artists and construction professionals who work with epoxy- and are chest freezer cold plunge enthusiasts. Because of the complexity involved, I strongly urge beginners: *do not* to use epoxy on your chest freezer! There are too many things that could go wrong.

If you want use epoxy, hire a professional. Your end cost with materials and labor could range from $500 - $1,000. There are two things to keep in mind:

1. It might take months to off-gas the strong odor. For some people this made their chest freezer unusable.

2. Use plant-based products that are non-toxic. Two brands suggested by an experienced epoxy person (who is also a member of our Facebook group) are Entropy Resins and Ecopoxy. I have not used either one, and they are included for reference only.

PRODUCTS TO AVOID

There are many other sealants on the market, including adhesives, glues, marine tape, paints, roof sealants, and several "As Seen on TV" products such as "Flex Seal." None of the Flex Seal line or products are suitable for sealing or lining your chest freezer.

Don't use them!

I dismissed most of them after learning just a bit more about them by reading the directions for use and application or the

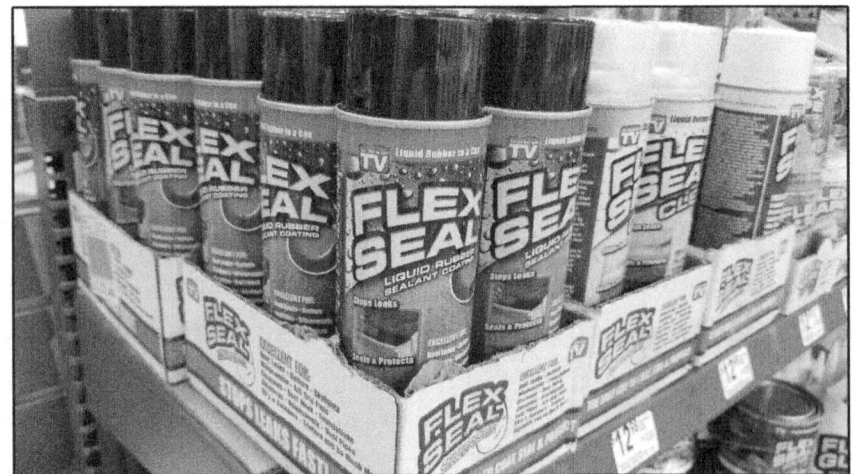

Do not use Flex Seal on your chest freezer

Manufacturers Safety Data Sheet (MSDS). I've also seen a number of problems reported from people who have used these products. Finally, after a few emails with their customer support team, it was officially declared "unsuitable."

I'm not discouraging you from using other products, but be cautious. If you find a different product, do your homework!

- Call the manufacturer directly and tell them that you want their advice on using their product for prolonged submersion in cold water and find out what they tell you.

- Tell them the chemicals or devices you will use for water sanitation and find out if they are compatible.

The single decision that led to a Pandora's Box of issues in my chest freezer journey was applying marine-grade waterproof tape to seal my seams. The tape had an intense chemical odor, which gave me a headache. Even after a few weeks of sitting in the sun, the smell did not diminish.

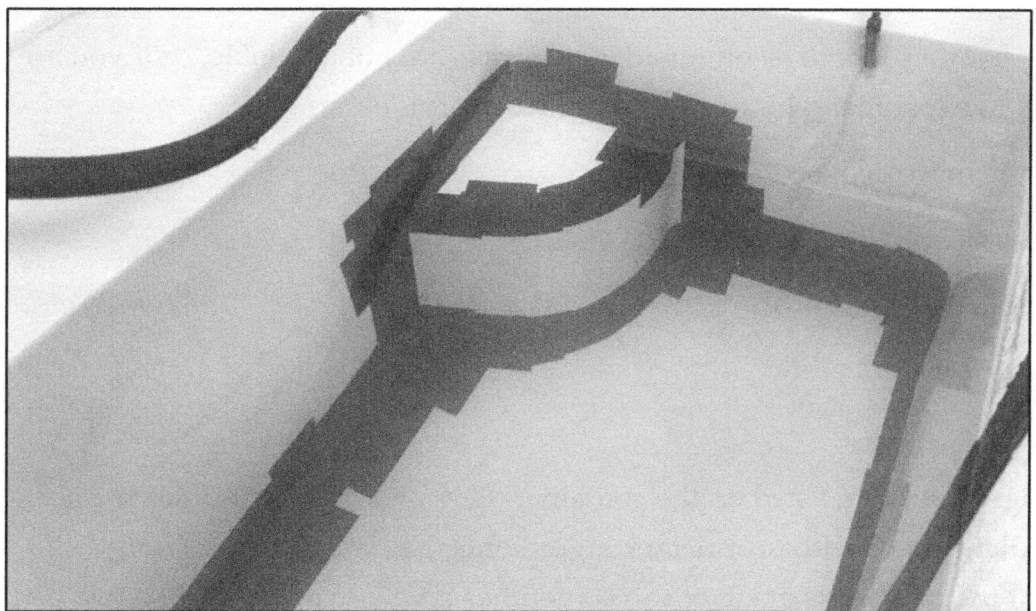

Marine tape – not recommended!

When I attempted to remove it, I quickly learned that it would not peel off easily. A small metal paint removal tool did not work either. So, I bought a heavy-duty scraper and while using that, accidentally gouged a hole through the wall. What

---

happened next is another story, but did provide me with useful information about the problems with using marine tape.

Tape Update

I recently found some marine tape that is advertised to be VOC free. If you are open to experimenting, you're welcome to try it out and let me know how it goes. However, at the time of publication, there are no *long-term* reports from anyone who has used marine tape.

As of October 16, 2019, one person on our Facebook group has reported 4-months of success with Gerband 586 Airtight Tape with no leaks or odors.

■ EXPLORING OTHER OPTIONS

One of the most common questions / posts in our Facebook group is someone asking about a new product they found to seal or line their chest freezer.

In most cases, a bit of research will determine that the product is unsuitable.

If you live in a country where recommended products are not available, or if you are feeling the call to experiment, here are a few practical guidelines.

1. Check the ingredients

2. Read product reviews

3. Review the Safety Data Sheet

4. Contact the manufacturer

Check the Ingredients

Usually the ingredients are listed on the container. However, I have found products with no ingredient list or with proprietary ingredients that are not disclosed. Knowing what the product is made of can sometimes give you a quick yes or no. Reference the ingredients with the compatibility charts in the appendices to ensure that your sanitation method will not deteriorate the product.

Read Product Reviews

Read the reviews on major retail sites such as Amazon. Do they have at least 70-80% 4 and 5-star reviews? What do the negative reviews complain about? Are there themes or patterns? Find out what users are saying on pool and hot tub forums about the product.

Review the Safety Data Sheet

Do a search for "product name" "safety data sheet." You will find information about the ingredients, toxicity levels, known problems, and risks.

Contact the Manufacturer

Go the manufacturer's website and find their contact information. Call or email them with the questions listed below.

Let them know that you are building a home-made cold plunge (or converting a chest freezer) and are researching products for waterproofing.

1. Is Product X a suitable liner for waterproofing the inside of the container / chest freezer? It will hold about 227-454 liters (60-120 gallons of water) and will be underwater for up to 3-6 months at a time.

2. Will Product X be OK with constant exposure to water temp. of 0-10 deg. C. (32-50 F)

3. Once it has dried/cured, is there any possibility of chemicals leaching into the water? I want to make sure that it is free of VOC's. My plan is to use the cold plunge 3-6 times a week and I need to ensure that there is zero risk of being exposed to any unsafe chemicals from the liner.

4. How long does it take for the product to cure?

5. After Product X dries/cures, how long does it take for any odor to go away?

6. Is Product X compatible with long term exposure to Epsom salt, chlorine, hydrogen peroxide, ozone, and UV lights?

When I contact manufacturers, I ask them all about all of the common sanitation methods because I'm looking for products that will work for all (or most) people. You may have your sanitation method selected, however, that could change for a number of reasons. Because of this, it's best to find a product that will be durable with the various options.

Be patient. Sometimes the "support" people are knowledgeable and helpful, and sometimes they are not. If you get a generic response with sales or marketing information, find out if there is a product manager or technical support person you can talk with.

Real World Setup

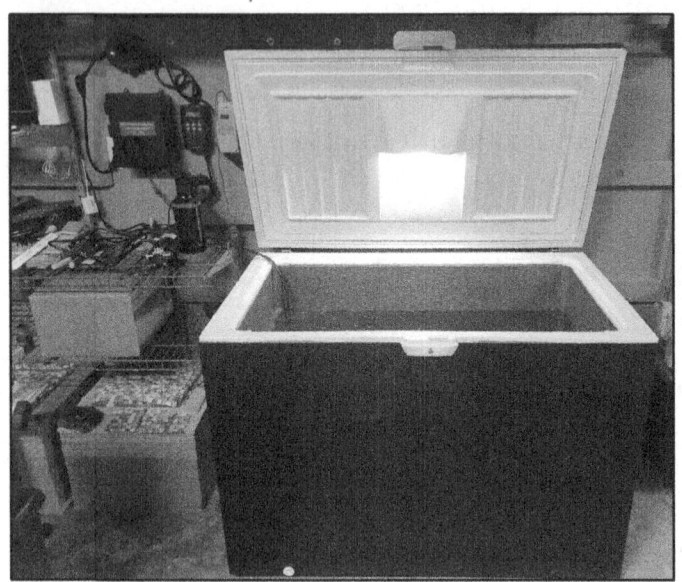 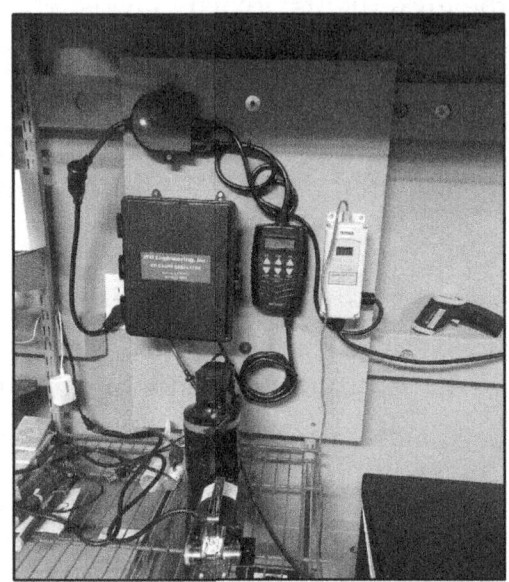

Chest freezer setup by Gordon Davis, USA

Whirlpool 14.8cf chest freezer:	$430
Line-X Premium Spray Liner inside and out with blue interior:	749
JED 203 Ozone Generator:	270
Aqua Logic Temperature controller:	216
SumpMarine UTP Portable Transfer Water Pump:	54.98
Marineland Magnum Polishing Internal Canister Filter:	37.99
Food Grade Hydrogen Peroxide 1 gal.:	37.51
Ozone Test Paper:	34.99
Smart Socket Outdoor plug:	23.79
B-LINK 7-day outdoor Heavy Duty programable Timer:	16.99
Elekcity Lasergrip Digital laser Thermometer:	15.99
Total Project Cost	**$1,8870.00**

Notes

_____

_____

_____

_____

_____

_____

_____

_____

_____

_____

_____

_____

_____

_____

"*I don't want to make the wrong mistake.*"

Yogi Berra

Chapter 5:
Waterproofing with Liners

There are two different types of liners for your chest freezer: removable and permanent. Removable liners provide a cost-effective and straightforward way to get started. Permanent liners cost quite a bit more and need expertise and specialized tools to apply. Both types of liners fall into two groups: do-it-yourself and professionally installed.

If you use a removable liner, I still recommend sealing your chest freezer. If you plan to use a permanent liner, sealing your freezer is unnecessary.

Neither type of liner interferes with the chest freezer cooling the water.

REMOVABLE LINERS

There are two types of removable liners: standard pond liners and custom-made liners.

Putting a pond liner in your chest freezer is quick and easy. Opinions differ about whether you should seal your freezer if using a liner. It depends on your risk tolerance.

The main question to think about is, "What happens if the liner cracks, tears, or gets a pin-hole leak?"

If your chest freezer is sealed, it will be OK. If it is not sealed, it may take a while to discover the problem. By that time, your chest freezer may be damaged beyond repair. That said, it is up to you.

It may be tempting to use landscaping plastic or an inexpensive pond liner from a local hardware store; however, I don't recommend it. Different materials are used to make pond liners, and some work better than others.

The best overall material for strength, durability, flexibility, and long-term use is EPDM, which is a form of synthetic rubber. It holds up very well in cold water and has excellent resistance to ozone.

Pond liners come in different thicknesses, usually measured in the US in thousands of inches (mils). How thick does the liner need to be? 45 mils (1.1 mm) is a safe bet. Thicker liners are available but may be problematic to fold into your chest freezer. Thinner liners made from stronger material are available but do not fold easily.

Liners found in most hardware stores are not a good choice because they are too thin.

Here is an overview:

Material & Thickness	Notes
EPDM (Ethylene Propylene Diene Monomer) 45 mil (1.1 mm)	<ul><li>Tear, puncture, and UV resistant.</li><li>Heavier than other products</li><li>Rated "A-Excellent" for ozone use, and salts</li><li>Not compatible with chlorine</li><li>Up to 20-year warranty</li><li>15' x 20': $195</li><li>Strongly recommended.</li></ul>
HDPE (High density Polyethylene)	<ul><li>Durable, but stiff; difficult to work with.</li><li>Not recommended.</li></ul>

Material & Thickness	Notes
LDPE (Low-Density Polyethylene) 40 mil (1 mm)	• Flexible but not as durable as other products • Rated "B-Good" for ozone use • 10-year warranty • 15' x 20': $170 • Not recommended
PVC (Polyvinyl Chloride) 20 mil (.5 mm)	• Shorter lifespan • Rated "B-Good" for ozone use • Rated "A-Excellent" for use with chlorine and salts • Warranty varies • 15' x 20' (457 x 609 cm): $165 • Recommended UNLESS you use a UV lamp
RPE (Reinforced Polyethylene) 20 mil (.5 mm)	• Because of its inflexibility, it is not suitable for being placed inside a chest freezer. The cost to make a custom insert is too high to be feasible. • Not recommended.

Most pond guys suggest putting a durable material underneath your pond liners to prevent punctures from rocks, roots, animals, and other things out in nature. While probably not necessary to add this underlayment to your chest freezer, it won't hurt.

A 5x5' (152 x 152 cm) piece of underlayment costs around $30.

CAUTION

Chlorine can weaken EPDM pond liners over time. Epsom salts are fine.

■ Sizing Your Liner

To buy the correct size liner, you'll need to know the interior measurements of your chest freezer.

Find the width, length, and depth.

My example uses round numbers to make it easy to follow.

Let's say we have a chest freezer with the following *interior* measurements:

Length: 4' (122 cm) left to right

Width: 2' (61 cm) front to back

Depth: 2.5' (76 cm) top to bottom

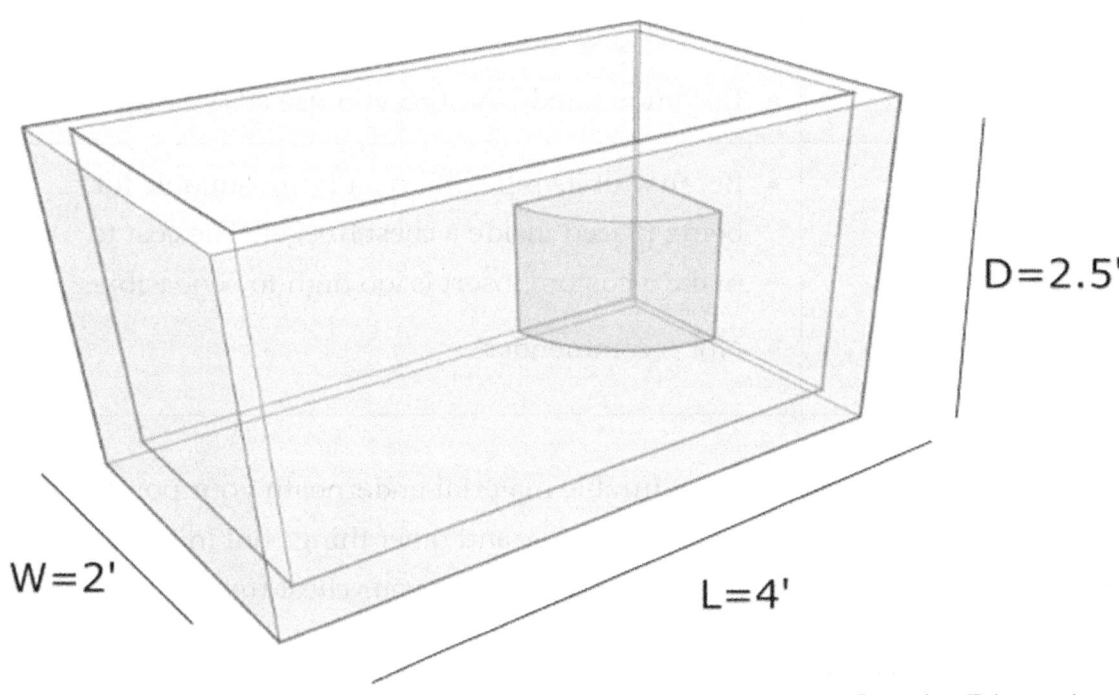

Interior Dimensions

Take your depth, multiply by 2, and add 2 feet (61 cm) for overhang. This would give you 7' (152 cm). Add that measurement to your width and depth.

In this example, you need a pond liner of 9' x 11', or 335 cm x 289 cm.

THE MATH

Imperial	Metric
2.5' depth x 2' = 5'	76 cm x 2 = 152 cm
5' + 2' = 7'	152 cm + 61 cm = 213 cm
Add 7' to the width and length.	Add 213 cm to the width and length.
4' length + 7 = 11	122 cm length + 213 cm = 335 cm
2.5' width + 7 = 9	76 cm width + 213 cm = 289 cm

Pond liners are typically sold in fixed sizes. In this case, you would need to round up to 10 x 15' (304 x 457 cm). It is better to buy a larger liner that you need to trim down than to have one that is too small.

Be sure to clean, or at least wipe off, both sides of your pond liner before you install it in your chest freezer.

■ Folding & Attaching Your Liner

It can be tricky to fold a pond liner into your chest freezer so it isn't bunched up. There are many ways to go about it. Here is one:

Find the middle of your liner and place it into the middle of the floor of your chest freezer. Fold in the corners as neatly as you can and make sure the liner overlaps the top of the walls and down onto the outside sides.

One great suggestion is to put heavy boxes on top of the pond liner on the chest freezer floor. This helps keep it in place and makes it easier to fold the sides.

Another way to make the liner easier to work with, and to fold around the edges is to use a heat gun. Cut a small piece off the corner of the liner first to experiment. The

---

heat makes the liner more pliable, but too much can melt the material. Use the lowest setting. Decent quality heat guns range in price from about $16 - $35.

■ Trimming the Liner

After the liner is in place, trim the liner around the handle/lock and the hinges on the back.

What do you do with the excess liner?

There are several options:

- Hang it over the edges

- Fold it up over the top of the closed lid

- Trim and tape it to the top or outside of the chest freezer walls

- Use a tie-down with a ratchet to secure it to the outside wall.

I recommend draping the liner over the top edges because that reduces the chances of water getting between your liner and the inside walls of your freezer.

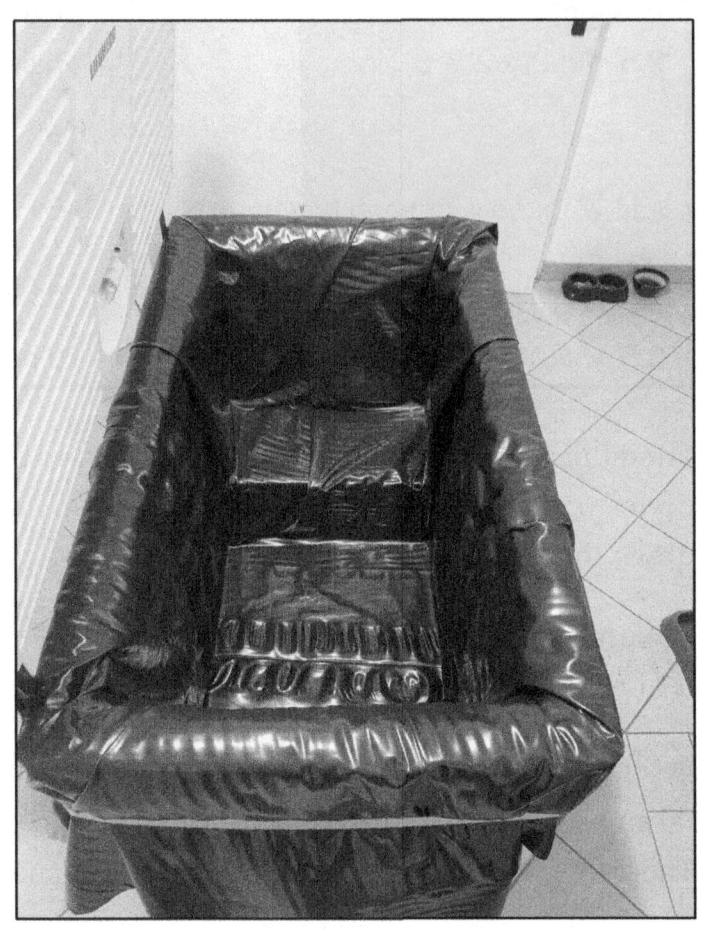

Liner with ratchet strap
Photo courtesy of Max Milian
Bucharest, Romania

If you use tape or a tie-down, secure it as close as possible to the top of the outside wall. The reason for this is that the top few edges of the outside walls should stay cooler because chiller lines do not run behind them. On my Whirlpool 15 cubic foot chest freezer, the top 2 - 3 inches remain cool. The less material you have touching the part of the walls that gets hot, the better.

Another option is to neatly trim the pond liner and put the tape on the top walls. Some people have used white tape so that it blends in with the molding on the chest freezer.

Do not tape the folds of the liner inside where it gathers in the corners or the walls meet the floor because that makes it difficult to remove and clean liner.

Use standard masking tape, which is easily removed. If you use marine adhesive tape, it can be very difficult (or impossible) to remove. Be careful to use tape that does not have a strong chemical odor.

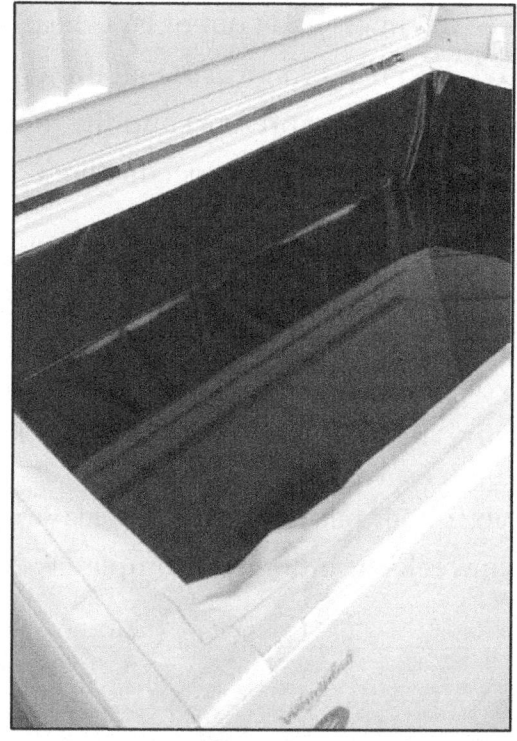

Liner with white tape on the top of the walls

■ Custom Made Liners

If you don't want to deal with all of the folds of a standard pond liner, you can have a custom liner made. I used a company called PolyFabrics (www.polyfabrics.com), but there are others.

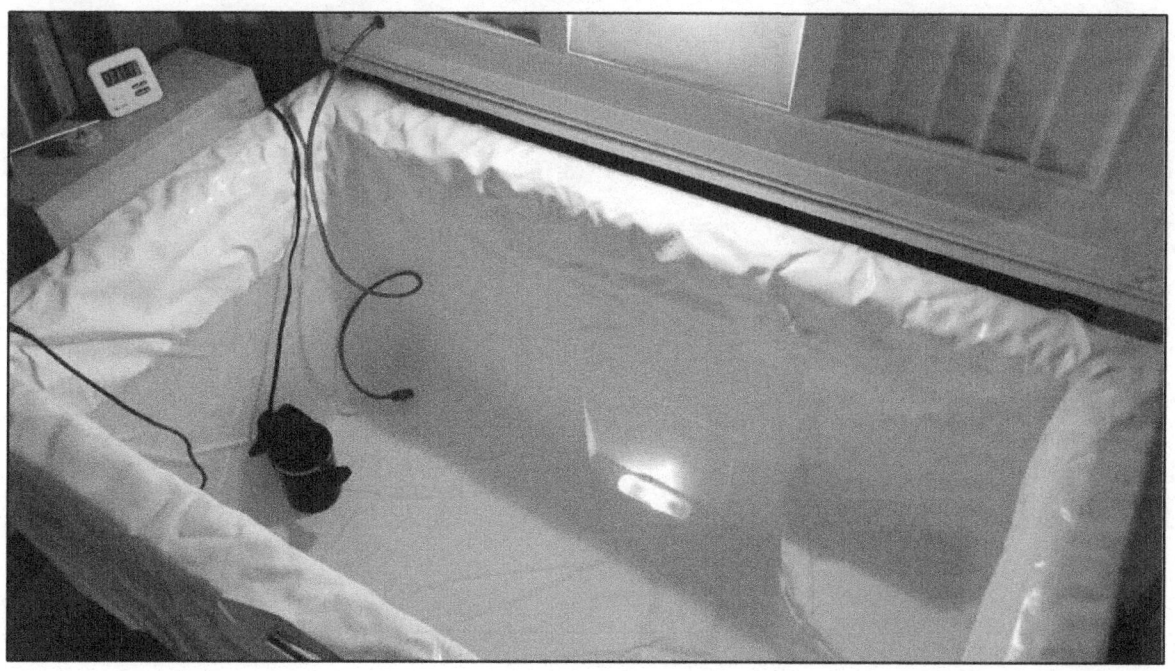

User-installed custom liner made from PVC

Have the liner made out of PVC because it has better compatibility with ozone than vinyl. You need to measure all dimensions of each surface inside (including the area covering the compressor) and the tops of the walls. Send them a drawing, and they make the liner to your specifications.

You can have them make holes for the hinges and the handle/lock – at an extra cost- or you can easily trim the liner around these areas with a pair of scissors.

If you have it in your budget, hire a professional who installs pool liners. He can ensure that the measurements are precise, as well as install your liner for you.

If your liner has a strong odor, leaving in the sun for a few days will help. It may take weeks or months to completely off-gas.

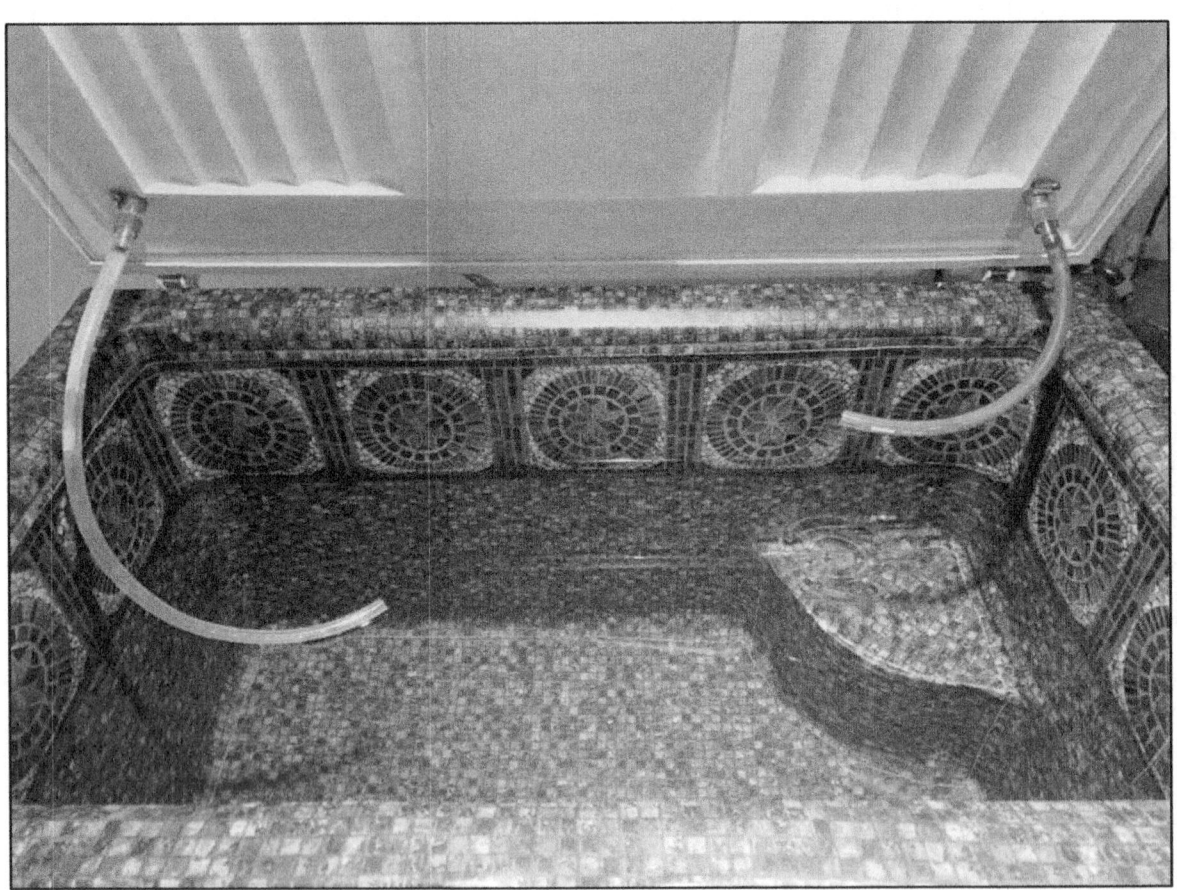

Darren E.'s custom vinyl pool liner, California, USA

Custom-made liners have a warranty that varies from one to twenty years. It might last longer than that, but the most significant risk is that the liner's seams may crack or separate and leak. This is why it's essential to seal your chest freezer seams (with JB Water Weld or high-quality silicone) even if you plan to use a removable liner.

Search the internet for "Custom pool liner" to find a company that will ship to your area. Having a pool professional do the measurements and install it can save you a lot of time and hassle. F

If you have installed a removable liner, the built-in drain in your chest freezer will no longer work. Refer to the section on draining your chest freezer for more information.

 PERMANENT LINERS

Most people are familiar with liners sprayed on to protect pickup truck beds. These liners provide a waterproof and durable coating.

There are two categories:

1. Do-it-yourself, and

2. Professionally applied

■ Do-It-Yourself

DIY permanent liners are made of rubber, epoxy, polyethylene, or other materials. The cheap ones come can be sprayed from their can or applied with a roller or brush. The better liners need a compressor and specialized equipment to be sprayed.

One huge issue with spray liners is that the chest freezer must be correctly prepared or the liner will not bond to surface. If you have bare metal (aluminum) walls and floor, this won't be as much of an issue, but you may need to apply a primer.

If your chest freezer has painted walls, you are in for a lot more work.

The hundreds of complaints in swimming pool and hot tub forums regarding failed DIY spray liners are one reason I don't recommend them.

Here are a few other issues and concerns:

- If you have a chest freezer with a painted interior, all of the paint must be removed and the metal walls thoroughly cleaned. There are many ways to do this, some better than others. The paint applied during the manufacturing process is durable and difficult to remove. Yes, my neighbors probably thought I was running a meth lab.

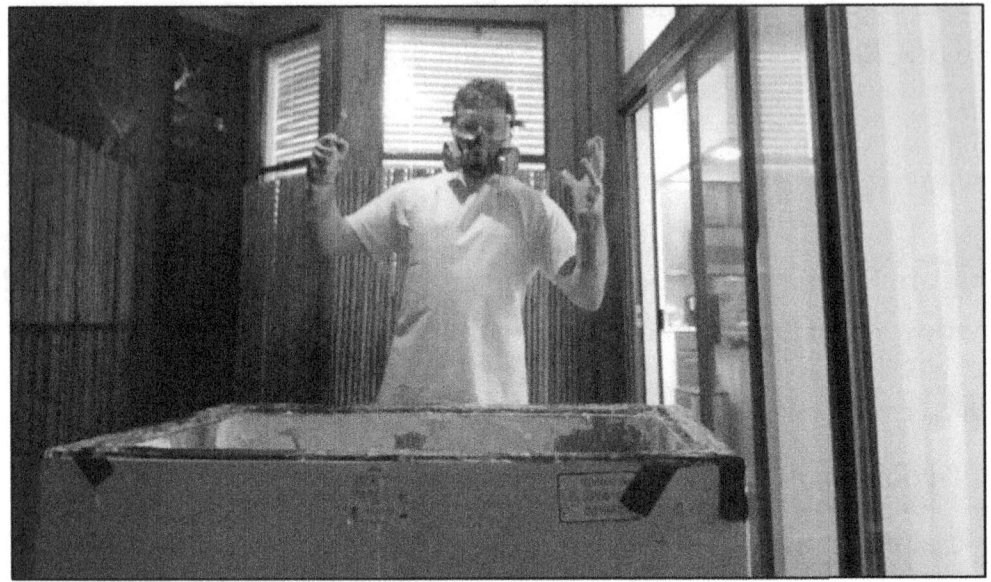

Protective gear for paint removal

- Mixing the chemicals for the spray liner can involve tricky timing.

- Some of the products can be difficult to apply correctly on vertical surfaces.

- There is a concern about toxic chemicals leaching into the water.

- The strong odor of some of the chemicals may take a very long time to dissipate (12+ months).

- Most of these products are not compatible with ozone, especially the surfaces exposed to air.

- The DIY spray liners that have a higher chance of working are expensive ($400 - $600+).

- Some of the better products are only available in large quantities costing thousands of dollars.

- If you are not familiar with using the equipment or working with these types of materials, there are countless mistakes that can cause the product to fail.

I found a DIY spray liner that was VOC-free and approved for potable water supplies. The materials alone cost about $400. I did not consider the time and effort needed to strip the paint, which turned out to be a huge undertaking.

I used simple scrapers, eco-chemicals, industrial solvents, paint removers, belt sanders, and muriatic acid. Working nights and weekends, it took so long for me to remove the paint that the exposed walls started to rust because of the humidity!

As an interesting side note, after all of the above abuse, the JB Water Weld is *still* on all of the seams! This is one of the reasons why I'm convinced it is a durable product.

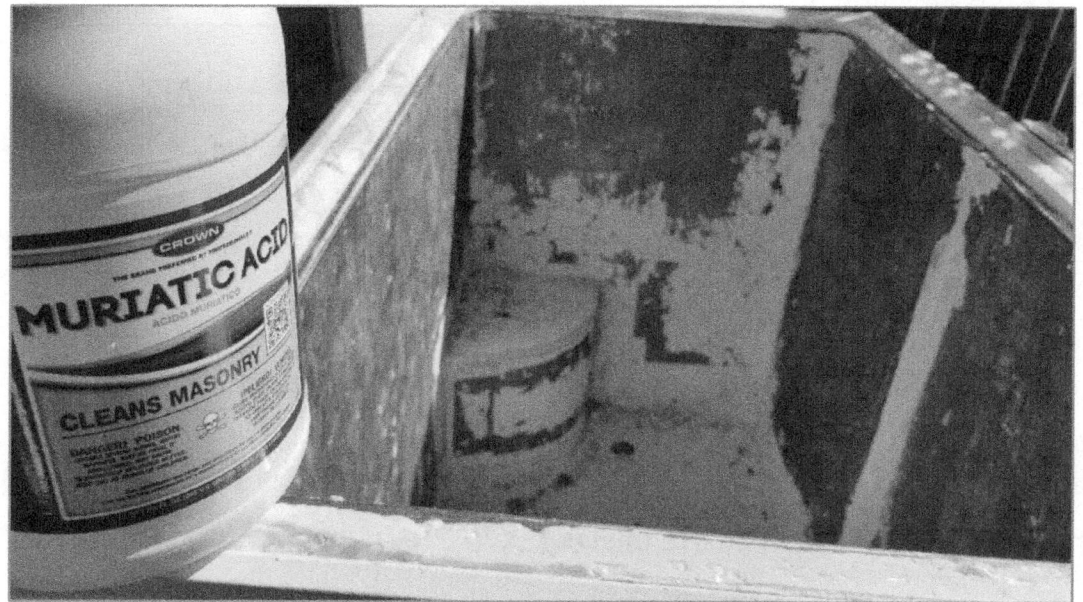

Stripping the paint

While removing the paint, I accidentally cracked the plastic molding on the top walls of the freezer. It had to be removed and replaced, which cost $140. You can avoid this problem if you are careful.

After receiving the products and instructions, I learned that the mixing and timing of applying the various chemicals were more complicated than what I cared to take on. Not to mention that the spray gun they loaned me was a basic model without precise controls and still required me to rent a compressor.

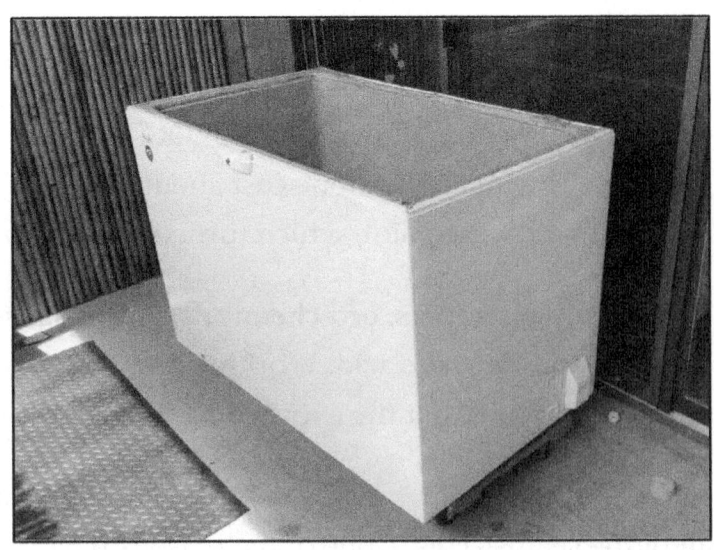

New DIY spray liner inside

Because of this, I hired an experienced professional with high-end equipment to apply it, which cost $450. After more than a year, I still have a slight smell in my chest freezer from the chemicals used to prep the walls. The biggest issue, however, is that ozone deteriorated the liner where it is exposed above the waterline. This grayish film looks terrible, is hard to clean, and

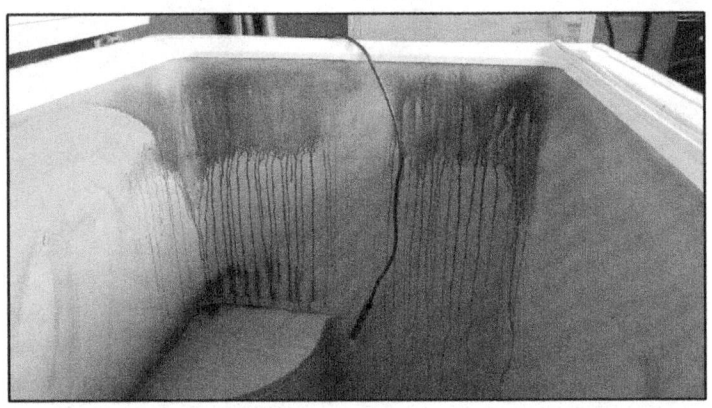

Deterioration of DIY spray liner from ozone

clogs up the filter. I made an expensive mistake.

Until I have substantial evidence to the contrary (which means reports from many users with 12+ months of use and no leaks), I do not recommend any DIY spray liner.

■ Commercial /Professional Liners

Professionally applied spray liners are great for a number of reasons. First is that someone else does all of the work. Second, you get a full warranty. The prices vary widely. I think they can be an excellent option if you have $400 - $1,500 in your budget.

In addition to sealing the inside of your chest freezer, you could also have the spray liner applied to the outside, (skipping the compressor equipment and vent areas), which would prevent scratches and dings and make your chest freezer bullet proof.

There are other benefits to having a permanent spray liner applied by a professional:

- They are 100% water-proof

- The top tier (premium) products are VOC free

- The premium options are UV and ozone resistant

- They have no thermal properties and don't interfere with the cooling function on the inside walls or the heat dissipation on the outside walls.

- They are super-durable and will outlast the components on your chest freezer. Some spray liners are used by the military on body armor and armored vehicles, and can even withstand explosives. There is an entertaining MythBusters episode on this.

- They can have a lifetime warranty

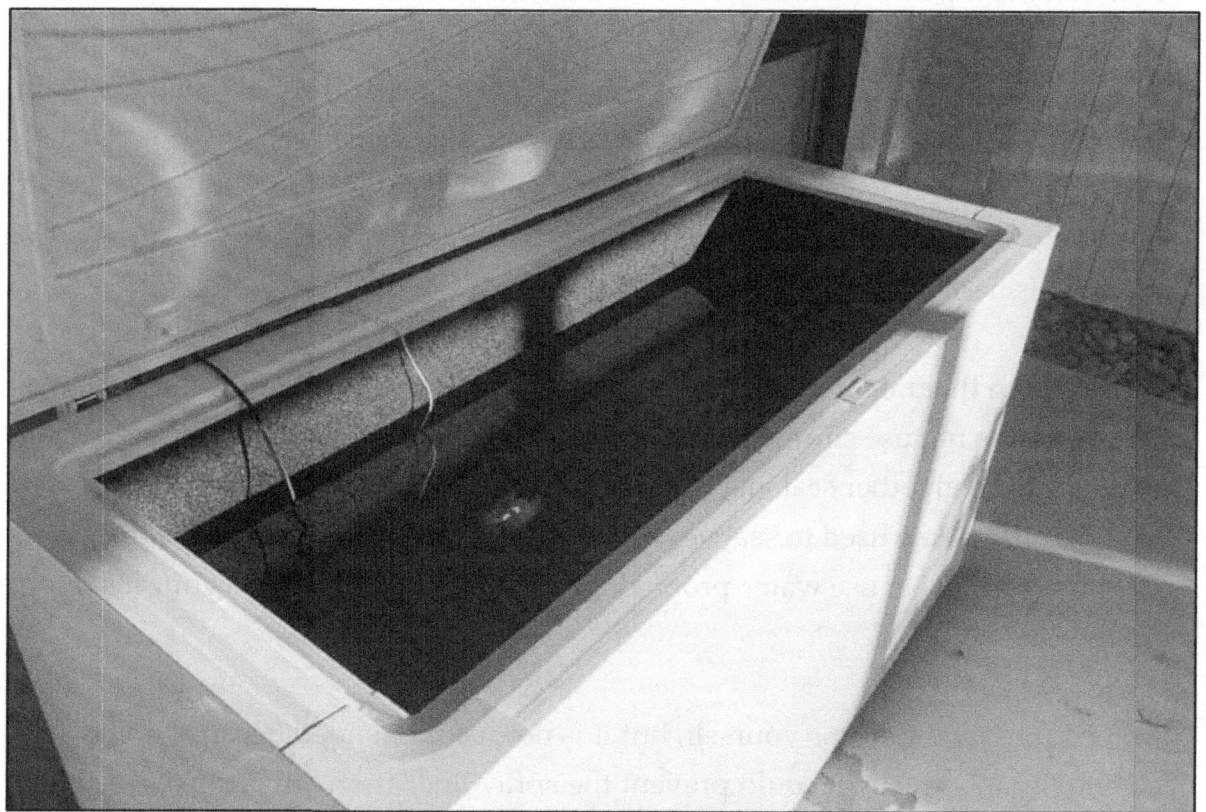

Garrett Ratner's Frigidaire with Platium Line-X, Dallas, TX.

As awesome as these products are, they are not without a few potential issues. Here are some things to keep in mind:

1. **Liner thickness**

   Professionally installed products can range from 1/8 inch to 1/4 inch (3.1 - 3 mm) thick, which could interfere with the lid closing or sealing completely. It should not be an issue if the liner is not too thick, or if the hinges on your chest freezer are adjustable (most are not). If you are uncertain, get the specs from your installer first and place temporary material of the same thickness around the trim to find out if the lid will still close and seal.

   It is strongly recommended to apply the liner on the plastic trim on the top wall.

2. **Sealing the seams prior to applying the liner**

   There is conflicting information about sealing the seams, and we are still figuring out what works best. Out of six chest freezer Line-X applications that I'm aware of, only one has had leaks. We believe it was because he did not seal the seam between the top of the inside walls and the trim.

   In a recent conversation with a Line-X franchise owner, he told me that any seam or crack must be sealed prior to Line-X being applied. This probably holds true for other brands as well. The dealer should include this as part of their bid, but be sure to ask them about it. There is conflicting information about what type of material is best.

   I spoke with the trainer at Line-X corporate and he agreed that the seams should be sealed. Do not use silicone. He recommended a polyurea caulk for best results, although other sealants could work. Some of the dealers use urethan caulking (the same used to seal new windshields in cars), which works fine. It *might* be possible to use water-proof aluminum tape, but talk with your installer first.

   You could seal the seams yourself, but it is not recommended because if you do something incorrectly it could prevent the spray liner from adhering correctly. It could also interfere with work they may need to do to prep the surface of the walls and floor.

If you want to ensure that it the work is done 100% correctly have the installer include that as part of their bid.

3. **Correct preparation**

A considerable part of the success or failure of spray-lined products is the preparation of the surface before they are applied. Be sure to discuss the surface preparation in advance with the technician.

Depending on the type of liner, the existing paint might need to be removed. Some might think this would make a good case for buying a chest freezer with an unpainted material. However, I strongly suspect (based on many reports) that these units are low quality and should be avoided if possible.

4. **Service unavailable**

Since most spray liner businesses are independently owned (and may or may not be a franchise), it is up to the owner to decide if they will coat a non-standard product (like a chest freezer) or not.

Some of the dealers may not be willing to line a chest freezer. There are dozens of spray liner franchises where I live in Central Texas, and most of them I talked with got twitchy when asked if they would spray something out of the ordinary.

Me: "Can you spray line a chest freezer?"

Them: "That ain't a truck."

After seven calls, I found one Line-X franchise and one other business where the installer thought it was a pretty awesome idea.

5. **Warranty**

Some dealers or franchises may not offer a lifetime warranty. This is probably not a huge concern since the liner will likely outlast your chest freezer. However, you do want to make sure that they at least warrant the workmanship for 30-90 days, which should be enough time for you to ensure that it was applied correctly.

6. **Toxic Chemicals**

   Toxic Two professional liners that have VOC-free products are Rhino and Line-X. They offer different grades of applications. Their upper-tier products are made of materials which have a strong resistance to ozone and UV. With Line-X, this is their "Platinum" coating. The low-end and mid-tier products are not recommended. I would only use the Platinum coating from Line-X.

7. **Getting an estimate**

   You may need to bring the chest freezer to their place of business to get an exact estimate. When I was looking into this, my chest freezer was set up and working, so it wasn't urgent. However, estimates range from $800 -$1,500.

8. **Which liner is best?**

   There are a number of professional liner options out there. All reports that I have so far are from people who have used Line-X. Line-X corporate has been very responsive to answering questions. Right now, Line-X is what I recommend.

   People with trucks have great things to say about Rhino. However, as far as I know, nobody has used it for their chest freezer.

9. **Which Line-X product should I use? What is the difference between them?**

   Line-X has a number of different products. I strongly recommend Platinum.

   The *standard product* (XS-100) is a blend of polyurea with polyurethane. This makes is a less durable product, which will discolor over time. Water will be very likely to seep through it within 8-10 years. That is based on data from trucks. Under constant submersion and cold temperatures, it is likely to be less than that.

   The product is not UV stable, so sunlight can cause it to deteriorate.

   The *premium product* (XS-350) is more robust, being 100% polyurea. It meets standards for potable water containers. However, it is also not UV-stable.

   The *platinum product* (XS-350) is the same as the premium product, but with an added topcoat, which will help it hold its color over time and provide UV resistance.

10. Texture

One other thing to consider, which may not be a big deal, is that the commercially applied spray liners do have a texture to them. In some, the level of texture can be varied, but it can't be left out. You won't have the smooth surface like in a hot tub or painted chest freezer.

11. Color

Standard bed-liners come in black. Many other colors are available, but usually add more to the cost. The downside of using black, or darker colors, is that it makes it difficult to see the quality of your water with a quick glance. With lighter liner colors, you can see quickly if your water is turning cloudy or has things floating in it that should be scooped out.

Notes

_____

_____

_____

_____

_____

_____

_____

_____

_____

_____

_____

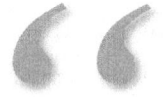 *Make everything as simple as possible,*

but not simpler.

Albert Einstein

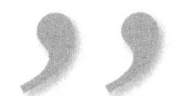

Chapter 6:
Supporting Your Freezer

The bottom of your chest freezer does not sit directly on the floor. Instead, four feet typically provide a small amount of elevation. The size and position of these feet can vary from one brand to another, but they are typically near the four corners, leaving most of the bottom unsupported.

Some people have reported that the floor of their chest freezer droops a bit under the weight of the water. While it is likely to be worse on the freezers with unpainted surfaces, I noticed the same problem on my chest freezer with painted walls.

This sagging can crack your seals and floors, causing leaks and other damage.

In this chapter you will learn a few different ways to reinforce your freezers' floors and walls

 HOW BIG ARE YOUR FEET?

Before you figure out what kind of support to use, you'll need to measure the height of the feet on your chest freezer and look at the bottom to see how it is constructed.

If there are castors or wheels on the bottom, see if they are easy to remove.

If the bottom of your chest freezer has different levels, measure from the largest area that is closest to the floor. You do not need to support any edges that overlap the main area

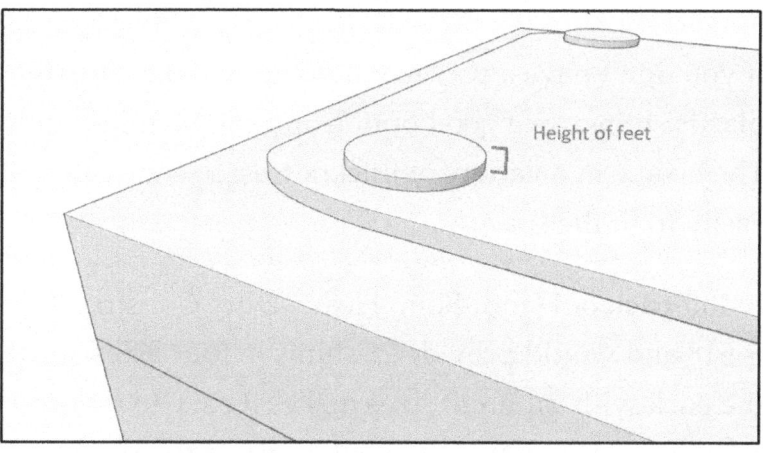

Feet on a Whirlpool

Measure the distance from the main outside bottom of the freezer to the floor. This distance is the height of the bottom supports.

There are a few simple options to support the bottom of your chest freezer.

One solution is to place a few shims under your chest freezer. Material that is water and rust-resistant is best, but just about anything substantial and dense enough works. Do not use shims thicker than the feet, or your chest freezer will not sit level to the floor. Be sure that the built-in feet still provide support.

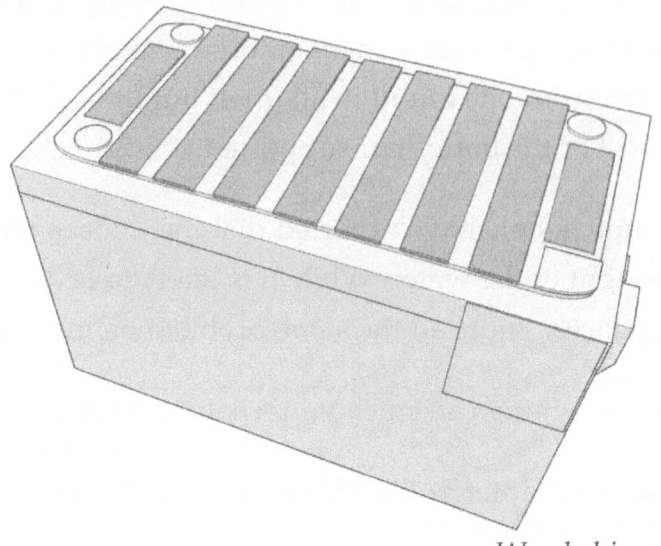

Wood shims

Wood Shims

Wood shims can be placed about 2 – 3 inches (5 – 8 cm) apart. Do not attach them to the chest freezer. Be sure that whatever you use will not scratch the paint on the bottom, which can result in the exposed metal rusting. Use pressure-treated (water resistant) wood for best results.

Plastic Shims

If you don't have a way to cut down wood to the right size, plastic shims are a good option and can be found online. They come in a variety of thicknesses, so they can be stacked easily to fit the space.

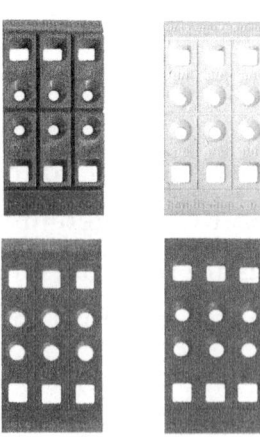

A 100-pack of Handi-Shim Heavy Duty Construction Shims is $18 and would provide 25 shims in four sizes. Ordering the pack with different sizes makes it easy to fix measuring mistakes and variances in the bottom of the freezer or your floor.

Handi-Shims

Stack the different colors of shims until you find the height that is needed. They are slippery and I suggest using duct tape to hold the stacked pieces together.

The picture to the right has 25 shims. Two packs would give better support. The closer they are, the more support they give.

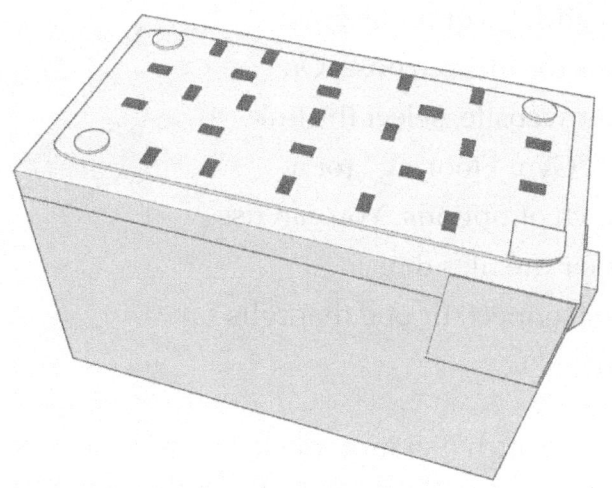

Plastic-- shims

Foam Tiles

The latest option I learned about is now my favorite. The plan is to use several interconnecting foam mats- the kind used for gym floors. Find a mat that is very close to the height of the feet. Make sure it is dense enough to provide support. If the mat is too squishy it won't help. Order the mats that are 2-feet (61 cm) square.

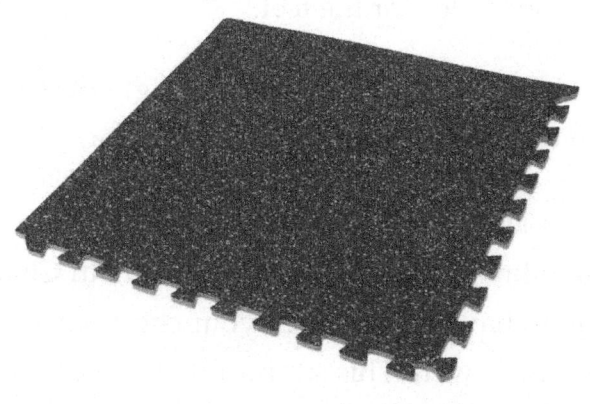

Foam tiles

"Engineering is the art of modelling materials we do not wholly understand, into shapes we cannot precisely analyse, so as to withstand forces we cannot properly assess, in such a way that the public has no reason to suspect the extent of our ignorance. "

-- Dr. A. R. Dykes, British Institution of Structural Engineers

GreatMats.com sells good mats for this purpose. On their website, select the link for "Gym Flooring" for a bunch of options. You can use either the tiles that interconnect, or one that rolls out.

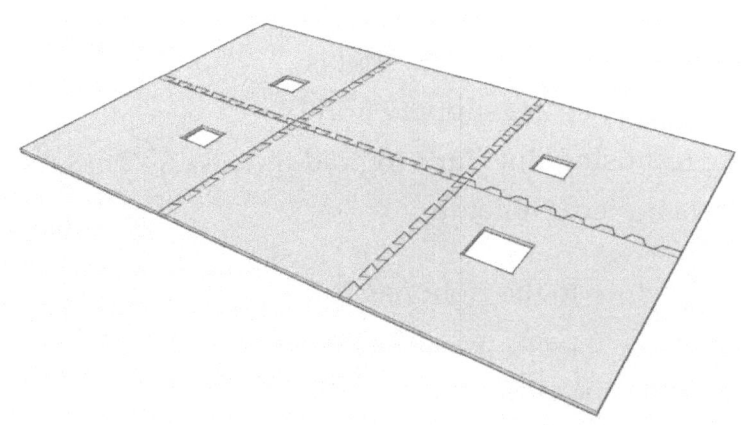

Connected tiles

The 3/8-inch (9.5 mm) thick mat is perfect for the Whirlpool Chest freezers.

Six tiles will cost about $40.

Cut four holes for the feet.

Again, be sure to measure the height of the feet on your chest freezer to ensure that you order the correct thickness of mat.

Spray Liners

Spray liners were discussed in detail in Chapter 5, but are worth mentioning here. If plan to have the inside of your chest freezer spray-lined, have them coat the entire bottom as well. This support will make shims unnecessary.

 ## OUTSIDE WALL SUPPORTS

Ratchet Straps

A number of people have reported that the outside seams or walls have bulged. If you are concerned about this, you could place one or two ratchet straps (tie down straps) around the outside walls.

If you have a professionally applied spray such as Rhino or Line-X installed on the inside of your chest freezer, no shims or straps should be needed.

Wet Area Floor Mat

A wet area floor mat protects the inside floor of your chest freezer. If the inside is unpainted, installing a mat is essential because the thin walls are easily damaged. If you have painted interior walls, a mat is still helpful (but optional)- especially if you have the outside floor supported.

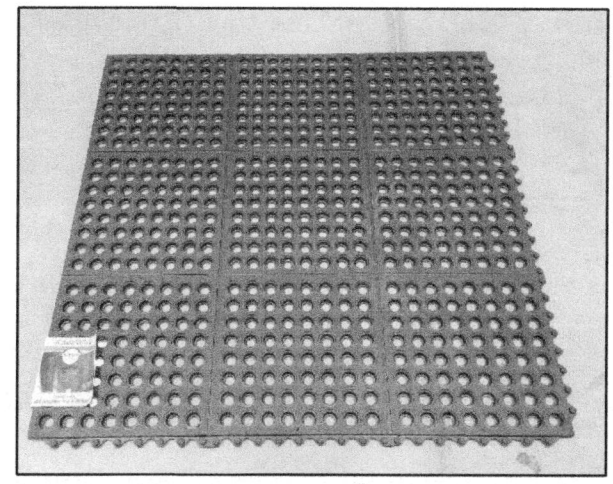

Wet area floor mat

Wet area floor mats can be found in a variety of sizes at hardware stores or online. If you can't find the correct size, cut a larger mat to fit.

They can range in price from $20 to $100+ depending on the size.

If you plan to use chlorine or ozone, make sure that the material is compatible.

Notes

_____

_____

_____

_____

_____

_____

_____

" *I have yet to see any problem,*
however complicated, which,
when you looked at it in the right way,
did not become still more complicated. "

Poul Anderson

Chapter 7: Accessories

Regardless of what setup you use, there are a few items that prove to be useful.

ESSENTIALS

1. GFCI plug or extension cord.

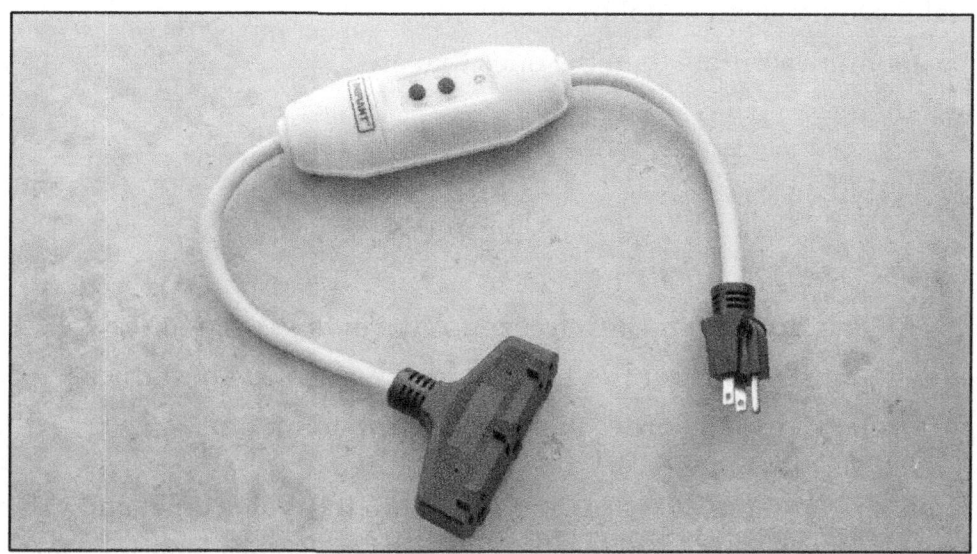

GFCI extension cord with three outlets

GFCI stands for Ground Fault Circuit Interrupt. If it detects a dangerous surge of electricity, the power shuts off immediately. The GFCI makes electrical devices safer around water.

Of course, you will always remember to unplug your chest freezer before you get in, won't you?

If you have a built in GFCI outlet, you do not need to add a GFCI extension cord.

$28

2. Thermometer

Use a thermometer to check your water temperature. This is a must for simple set-ups but also helpful with systems using temperature controllers to verify that the system works correctly.

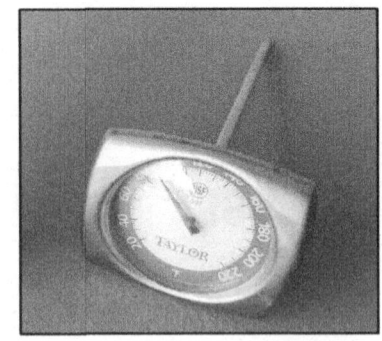

Analog thermometer

Buy an inexpensive analog meat or candy thermometer. If your budget allows and you prefer something fancy, you can use a digital thermometer. Digital thermometers with a sensor probe are more accurate than the ones that are infrared or touchless.

$6 - $10 for basic/$15 - $140 digital.

3. Garden Hose

A garden hose helps fill and drain your chest freezer. A drain to garden hose adapter is included with most new chest freezers. If you have a used chest freezer without that adapter, you can usually order the replacement online.

Cheap hoses work, but are far more likely to pinch and stop the water flow, and can be difficult to coil. If it is in your budget to buy a more expensive hose, you may be pleased with how much easier they are to use, coil, and store.

$15 - $60

4. Faucet to Garden Hose Adapter

If you live in an apartment or don't have access to an outdoor spigot, you can connect a garden hose to a standard sink faucet with an adapter. This item is available at hardware stores.

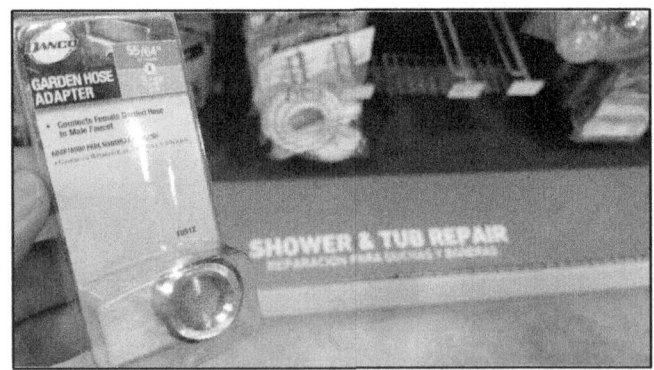

Faucet to garden hose adapter

Both faucets and garden hoses have different sizes of fittings. Be sure to purchase an adapter that fits.

$8 - $30

5. Pump or Siphon

If you plan to seal the hole of the drain or install a liner, you'll need a transfer pump or siphon to drain the water.

Good transfer pumps can run from $80 - $300

A hand pump siphon runs $10 - $20.

ELECTRICAL

1. Heavy-duty extension cords

GFCI extension cords I have seen are less than 3' (.9 meters) long. Adding a longer extension cord is helpful. Get a heavy-duty grounded extension cord made for workshops or power tools. I also find it helpful to have everything plugged into a single extension cord. This way, I only have one thing to unplug.

If you use a timer, you may need to have a short extension cord to go between the timer and the outlet.

$10 - $50 depending upon the length

2. Multi-outlet power strip

Depending on how many pieces of additional equipment you have in your setup, you may need a multi-outlet power strip. Get one that is weatherproof or water-resistant.

$20 - $40

▌NICE TO HAVE

The items listed here are optional but helpful.

1. Digital Countdown Timer
A countdown timer lets you focus on breathing and being present rather than worrying about how much time you have left.

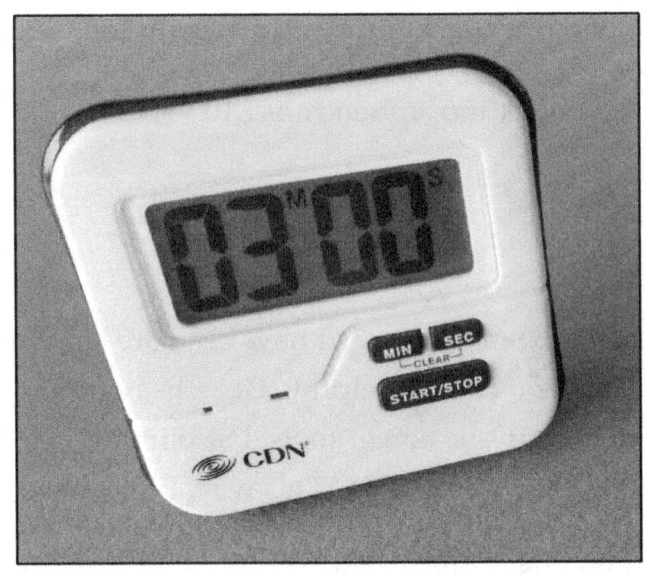

Digital countdown timer

Many people use their phone's built-in timer or download a cool app. However, having your phone near your cold tub is not safe – for you or the phone.

The timer pictured is the one I use, and I like that it is waterproof, has a stand and large numbers.

$10 - $15

2. One Small Step
Your chest freezer is more comfortable to climb into and out of with a small step. If you are tall enough, this may be optional, but still helpful.

Any sturdy (heavy duty) single step that is slip-resistant would work. A height between 6-9 inches (15 - 23 cm) is best. Some people have ordered steps designed for hot tubs. They usually come with two steps and are much wider than common step stools.

$15 - $75

3. Pre-Filter
Placing pre-filters on your garden hose will reduce sediment and chlorine.

■ MAINTENANCE

1. Fine Mesh Fish Net

No, not the stockings (unless you want to perform some freezer burlesque) - the net for scooping up fish! They are handy for scooping out stuff that you might see floating in your water.

Note: Do not put fish in your chest freezer.

$2 - $8

2. One-gallon / 4-liter bucket

A small bucket comes in handy for several things. It is good for emptying excess water in your freezer and can hold the fish net, or cleaning cloths.

$10 - $15

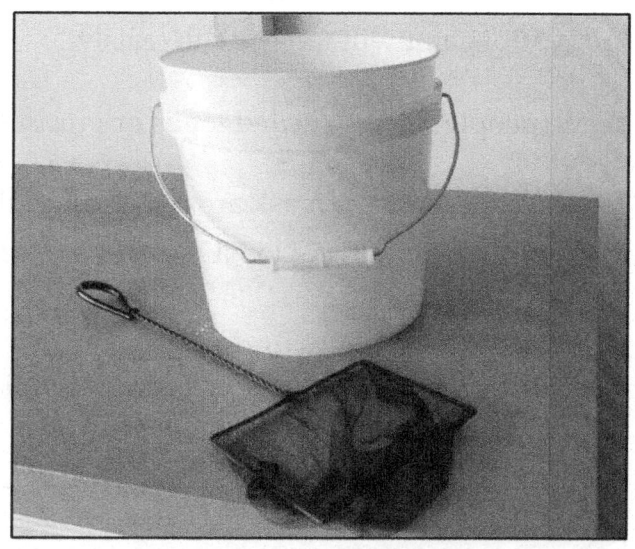

Fish net & small bucket

3. Cleaning cloth.

Keep a few small absorbable lint-free cloths around to wipe down splashes and condensation each time you use your chest freezer. I use different cloths for the inside and outside. I like microfiber, but any cleaning rag will do. If you dislike lint or cloths that snag, flat cloth baby diapers or burp rags are a good choice.

$5 - $25

4. Spa Vacuum

A manual or battery-powered hot-tub vacuum makes it easy to remove small debris and dirt. They can be found online or in local hot-tub supply stores.

$30 - $60

■ STYLING THE OUTSIDE

1. Painting

The outside of your chest freezer can be painted. Appliance epoxy spray paint holds up best if you plan to paint the entire surface. It is self-priming and can be applied over the existing paint. However, it is only available in a few basic colors (black, white, almond, and biscuit).

If you prefer a different color, you can use any standard spray paint, but it needs to be coated with a clear enamel gloss protective spray. If you don't use the protective spray, the paint will fade or chip easily.

Some people have stenciled logos or phrases on the outside for motivation.

Use painters' tape to mask around the handles, hinges, gaskets, and other areas that should not be painted. Do NOT paint any of the mechanics!

2. Specialty Wraps

Special wraps made from vinyl can be applied to your chest freezer. Standard and custom options are available.

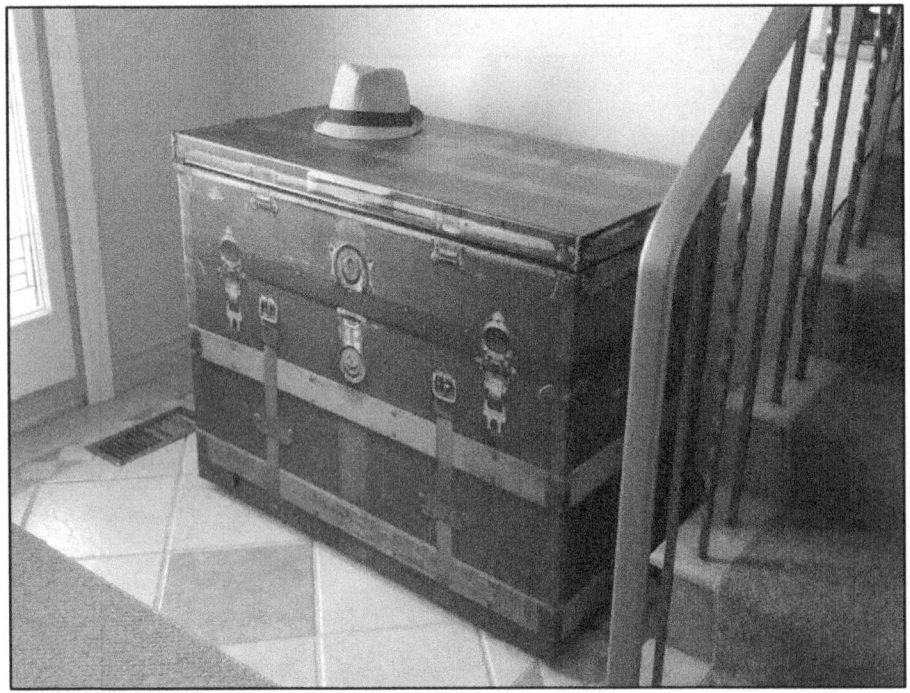

Vintage trunk chest freezer wrap from RMWraps.com

Notes

_____

_____

_____

_____

_____

_____

_____

_____

_____

_____

_____

_____

_____

_____

_____

" " *The odds of going to the store*

for a loaf of bread and coming out

with only a loaf of bread

are three billion to one.

Erma Bombeck

Chapter 8: Placement of Wires, Tubes & Other Equipment

Besides water sanitation, which is discussed in the next three chapters, there are two more issues to address before you start using your chest freezer:

1. What location is best for additional equipment such as ozone generators, and temperature controllers, and

2. What is the best way to connect the tubes, cables, and wires?

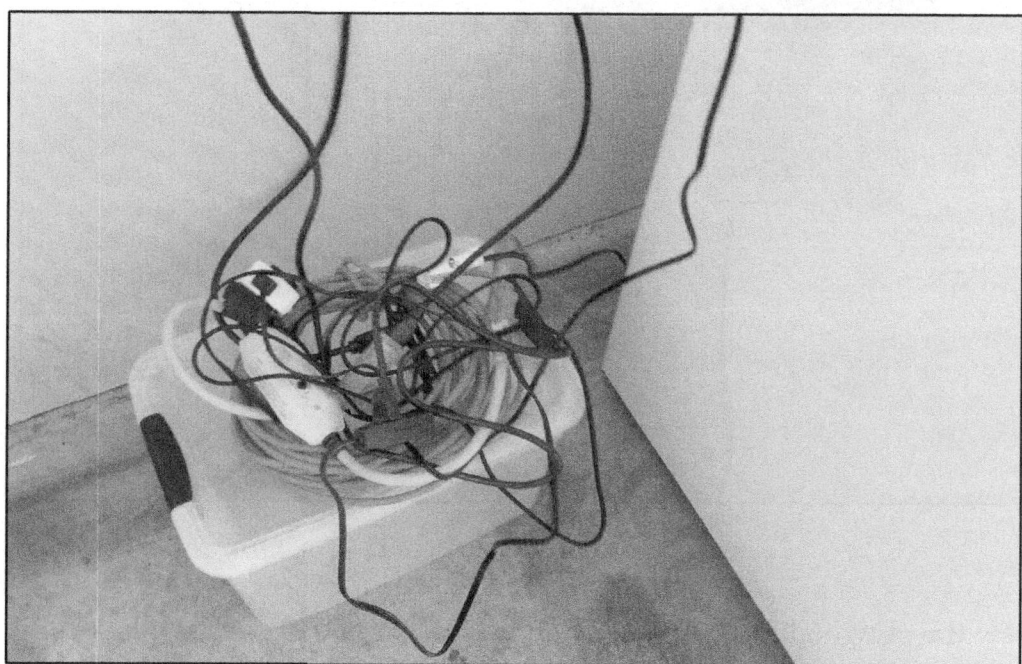

A plastic bin keeps these cables and wires off the floor

WALL MOUNTS AND SHELVES

Additional equipment can either be mounted to a wall or placed on a shelf. Some equipment, like the JED ozone generator, must be in an upright position to work correctly.

In the setup pictured below, my friend, Paulo, mounted a small piece of project plywood to the wall of his garage. He attached the ozone generator and temperature controller to that board.

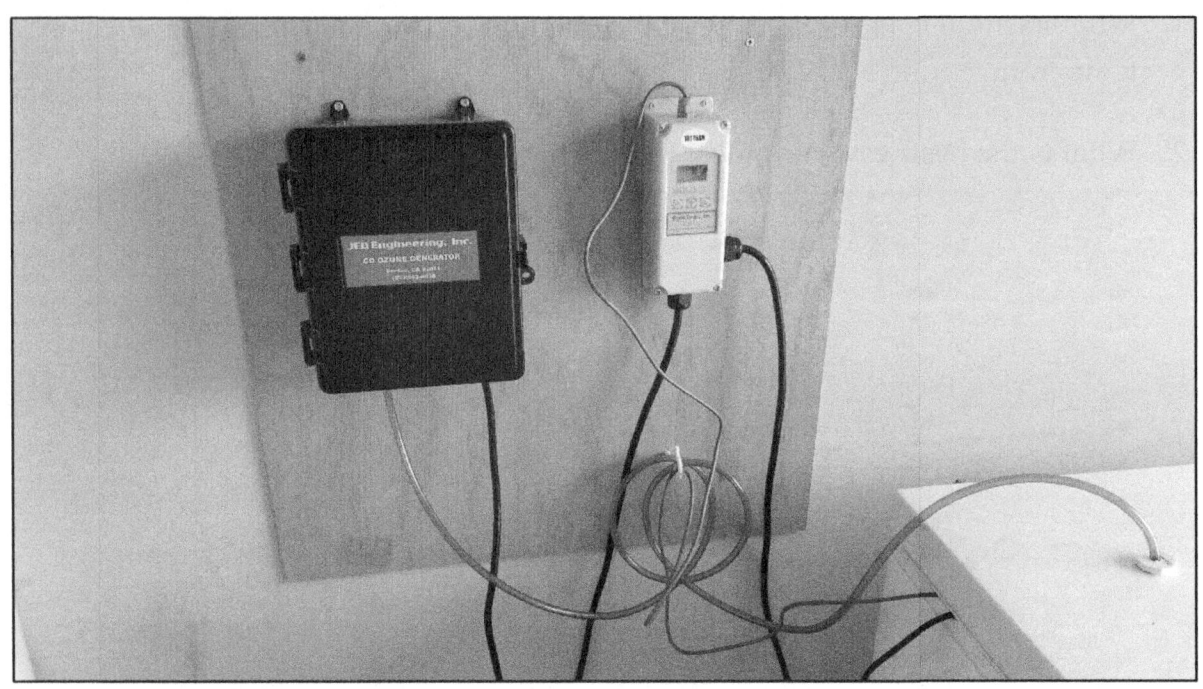

Wall-mounted project board

Be sure to screw the plywood into the studs behind the sheetrock so that it is secure. If you don't have or can't find studs behind the wall, use heavy-duty wall anchors.

Another option is to buy or make a shelf. Use water-resistant material.

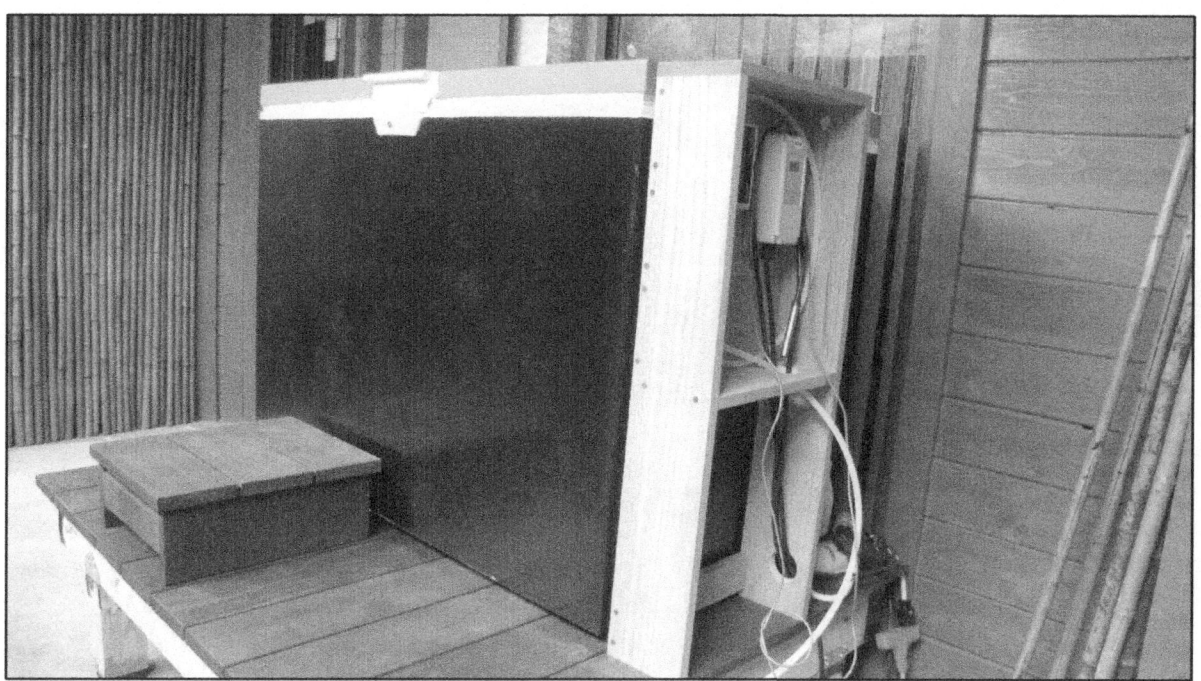

WIRES AND TUBES

There are only a few wires, cords or tubes that would typically go inside of your chest freezer:

1. Power cords (UV light, pump)

2. Sensor wires (temperature controller)

3. Tubing (ozone generator, external pumps)

Let's start with the easy ones: power cords and sensor wires.

Power cords are typically flat, and sensor wires are relatively thin. Because of this, it is straightforward to place them over the top edge of the freezer wall and close the lid over them without risk of damage.

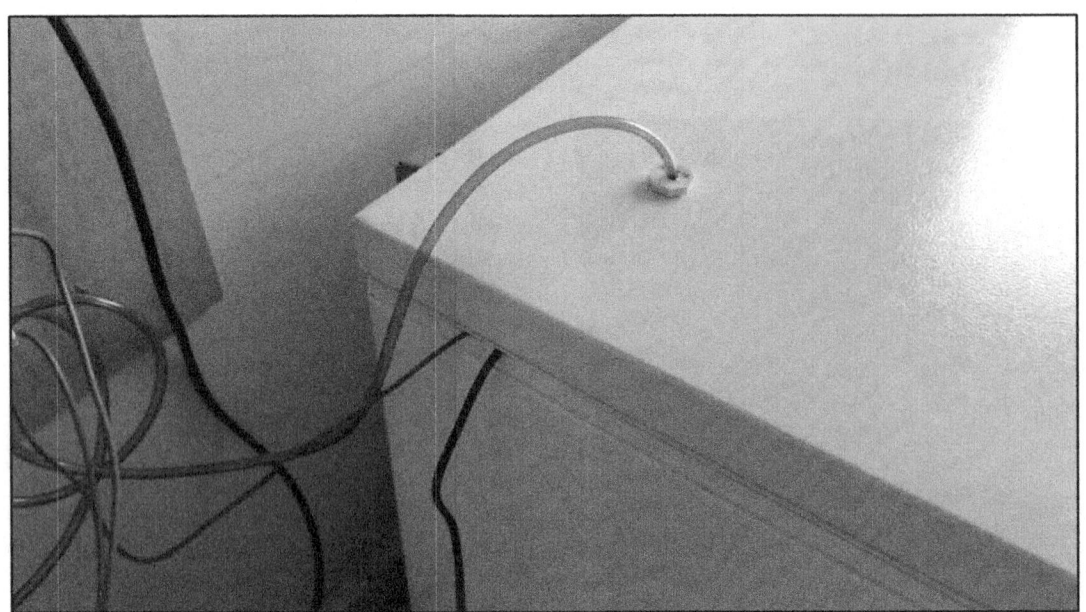

Pump power cord, temp. sensor, and ozone tube

It makes the most sense to place the wires or cords over the right or left edge of the freezer. If placed in the front of the lid, they would be in the way of entering and exiting. In the back, they have would be placed between the hinges and under the lid, making them hard to move and remove.

The ozone generator tube can be placed over the wall edge, but creates a gap, allowing warm air, dust, and bugs to get inside.

Power cords and sensor wires only create a tiny gap in the seal. You can fill this gap with foam rubber insulation or weather stripping.

It is a good idea to keep all of your cables and wires off the floor where they would be more likely to get wet.

CAUTION

Do NOT use spray foam to seal any gaps on your chest freezer.

It is possible to cut a small notch in the seal under the lid to better accommodate the ozone tube. Use caution. The inside of the lid is typically made of molded plastic hat may not have support or insulation behind it. Holes in this plastic might cause it to detach or incorrectly seal when closed.

▇ DRILLINGTHROUGH THE LID

Another option is to drill a hole in the lid. This requires a bit of skill with a drill, but it is not difficult.

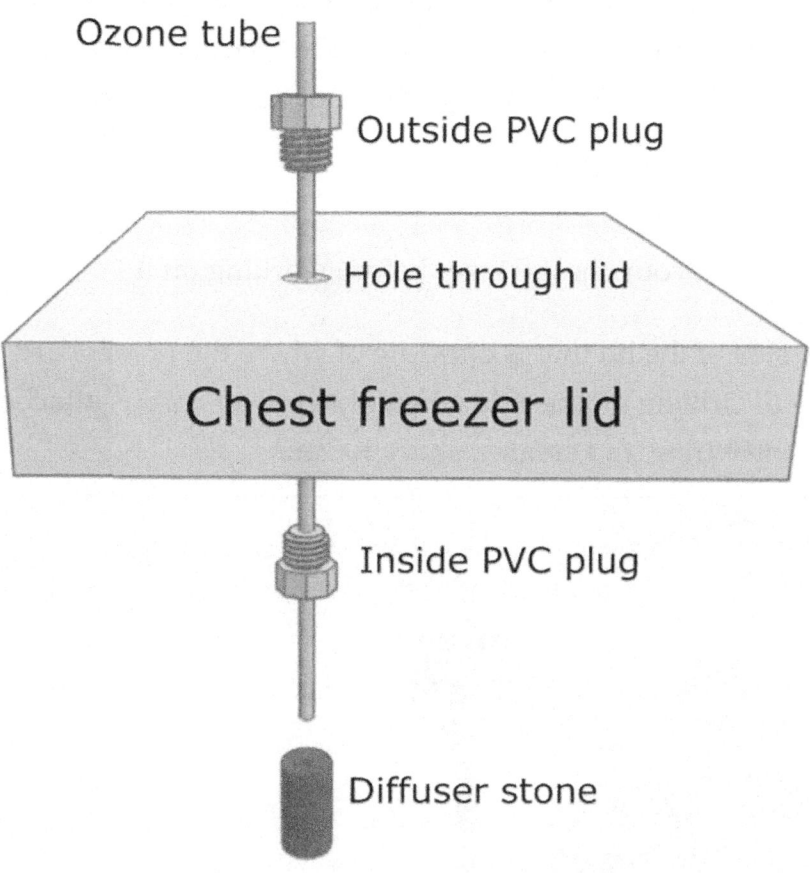

Ozone tube

Outside PVC plug

Hole through lid

Chest freezer lid

Inside PVC plug

Diffuser stone

Diagram of ozone tubing

I decided to run only the ozone tube through the lid, but you could go that route for all of your cables and wires. Here are the instructions for making a hole in the lid for 1/4" (.63 cm) ozone generator tube. The same steps apply for sensors or power cords. Measure the size of each object that will pass through the lid. Make sure that the PVC plug and the hole you drill for it is the correct size.

If you choose to put a power cord through the lid, you will either need to make a hole large enough for the plug end to fit through, or cut off the plug and replace it.

Equipment needed:

1. Power Drill

2. 1" (2.54 cm) hole saw

3. One 1/4" (.63 cm) drill bit (same size as the outer diameter of the tube)

4. Two 3/4" (.635 cm) threaded PCV plugs. The outer diameter of the threads on the plug need to be a tiny bit wider than the hole saw. Be sure to match the plugs to your hole saw by physical size, not just by description.

5. Small piece of rubber foam insulation.

Here are the steps:

1. Always unplug your chest freezer before working on it.

2. Find the side of the lid that is opposite of where the power cord for the light is attached. Drilling on the side where that power cord is attached may damage the wiring and create a shock hazard.

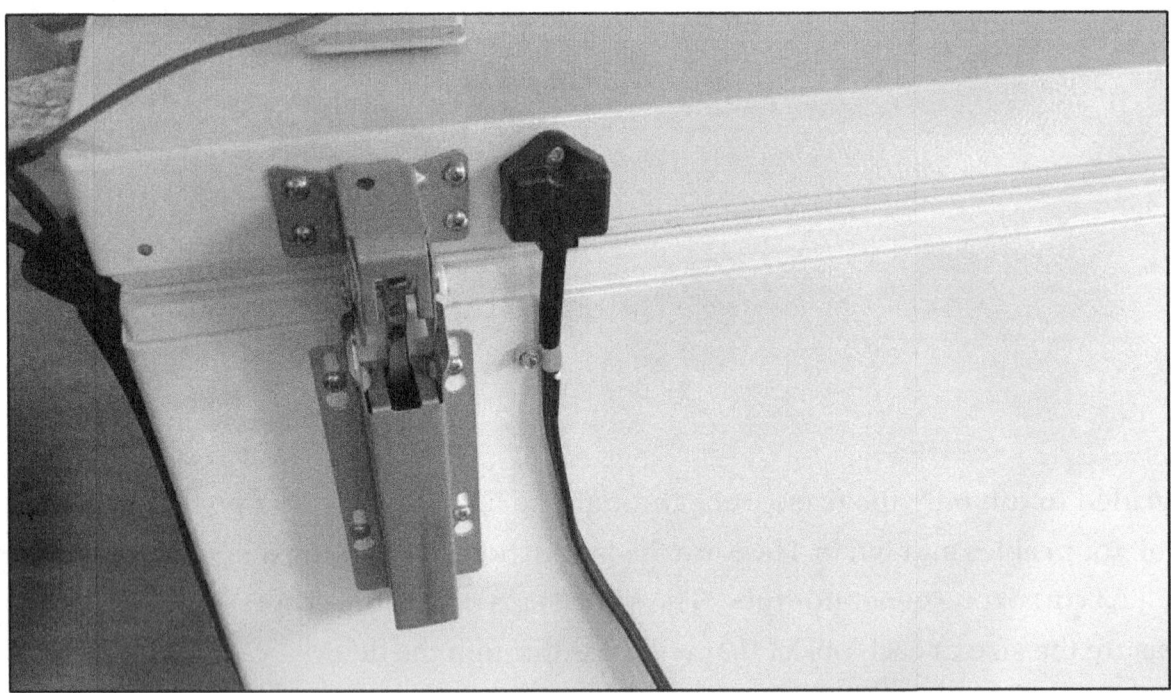

Avoid the side of the lid with the power cord

3. Open the lid and find a good spot:

    a. It should be toward the back, closer to the hinges, so the tube moves less when the lid is opened and closed. If you drill the hole toward the front, too much movement can damage the tube.

    b. Drill the hole at least 2 – 5 inches (4 – 5 cm) from the back inside of the chest freezer so that it won't interfere with the lid closing.

    c. If the inside of the lid has grooves or indentions, drill between them.

    d. Drill from either the outside in or the inside out. It doesn't matter either way. However, keep in mind:

        i.   Drilling from the inside makes it easier to position the hole correctly.

        ii. If you drill from the outside, have the lid open so that a friend can hold the plastic liner inside the lid to keep it from popping off. Be VERY CAREFUL to hold the lid AWAY from where the hole is drilled.

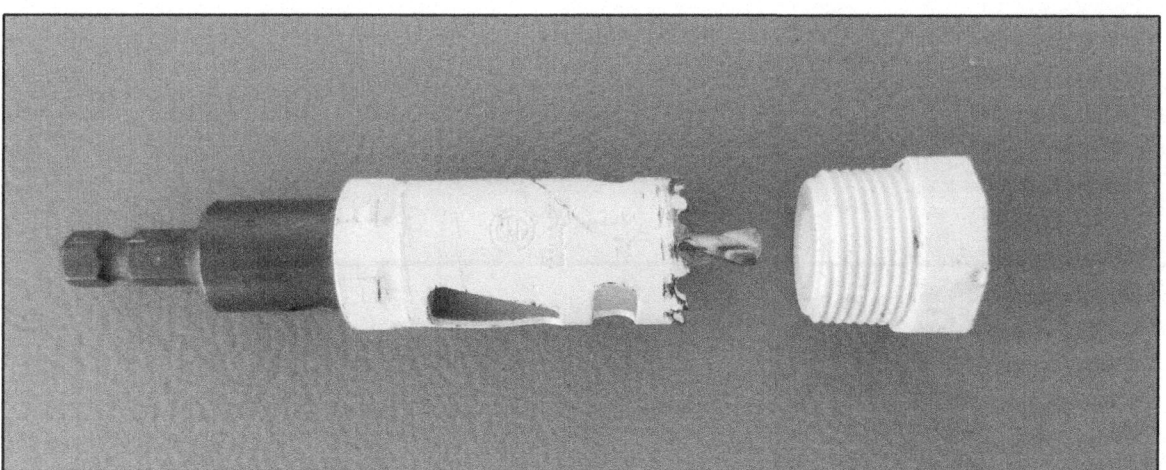

3/4" (.635 cm) Outer Diameter PVC plug and 1" (2.54 cm) hole saw

4. With the hole saw in place, have a friend hold the lid steady. Do not put pressure on the hinges.

5. Start drilling. When the hole saw has reached far enough inside the lid, the foam insulation fills it up and prevents it from going all the way through the top.

6. Stop drilling. Remove foam insulation from the hole saw bit.

7. Continue drilling until you go all the way through the lid.

8. Take the 1/4-inch (.63 cm) drill bit and drill a hole in the center of both threaded PVC plugs.

9. Thread the ozone tube through the top of one plug, the hole in the lid, and the bottom of the plug beneath the lid before you attach the bubbler stone and before you connect it to the ozone generator.

10. Turn the PVC plugs clockwise to the top outside and inside of the lid. They will not tighten completely. You are welcome to seal the plugs to the lid, but this is optional. They can be sealed with JB Water Weld or silicone. Seal only the outside edges.

11. Attach the bubbler stone to the tube. Make sure that there is enough tubing inside the chest freezer for the bubbler stone to reach close to the floor.

12. Cut small pieces of foam rubber insulation and insert them around the tube on the outside PVC plug. The foam secures the tubing and seals the hole. Do not apply sealants or adhesives to the PVC foam or the ozone tube!

UPGRADE OPTION

In the years following my initial setup, I discovered that a number of industrial cable pass-throughs and grommets are available that can be used in place of the modified PVC plug. Some of them are water and air-tight, which would be great for our application. However, at this point I have only researched these options, and have not used them in practice. The prices I have seen range from $5 to $30 per grommet / pass through.

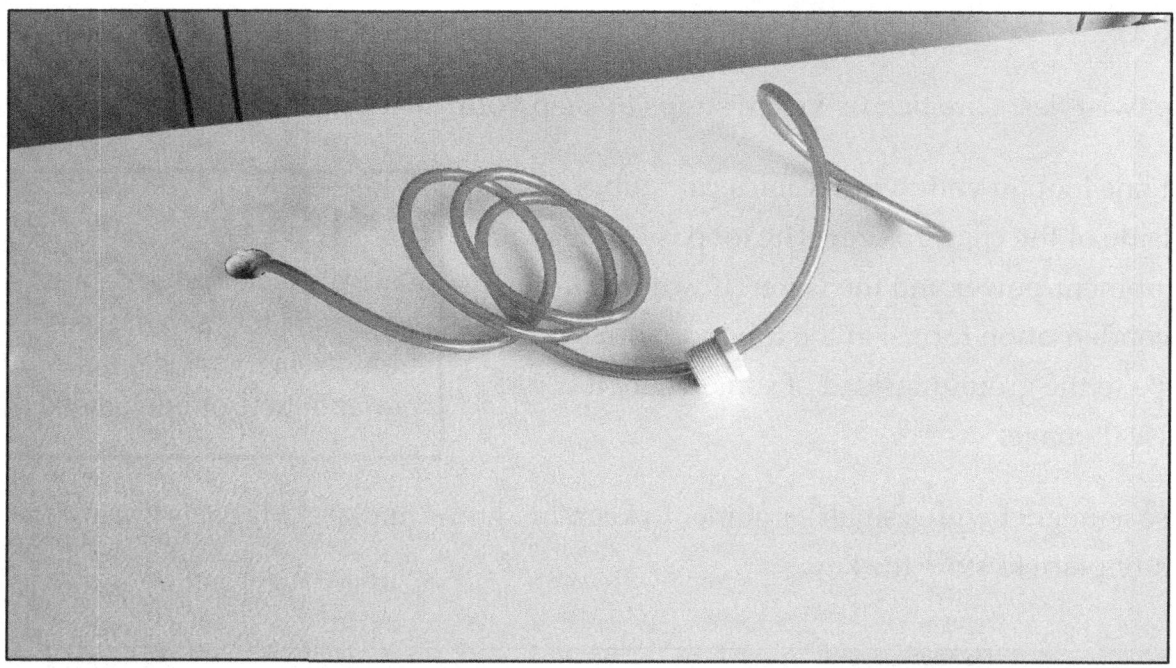

Hole with tubing and PVC plug

Note: The picture below shows two PVC plugs in the lid. This was for an early setup that had an external aquarium pump and filter. The second plug is now unused and has been sealed.

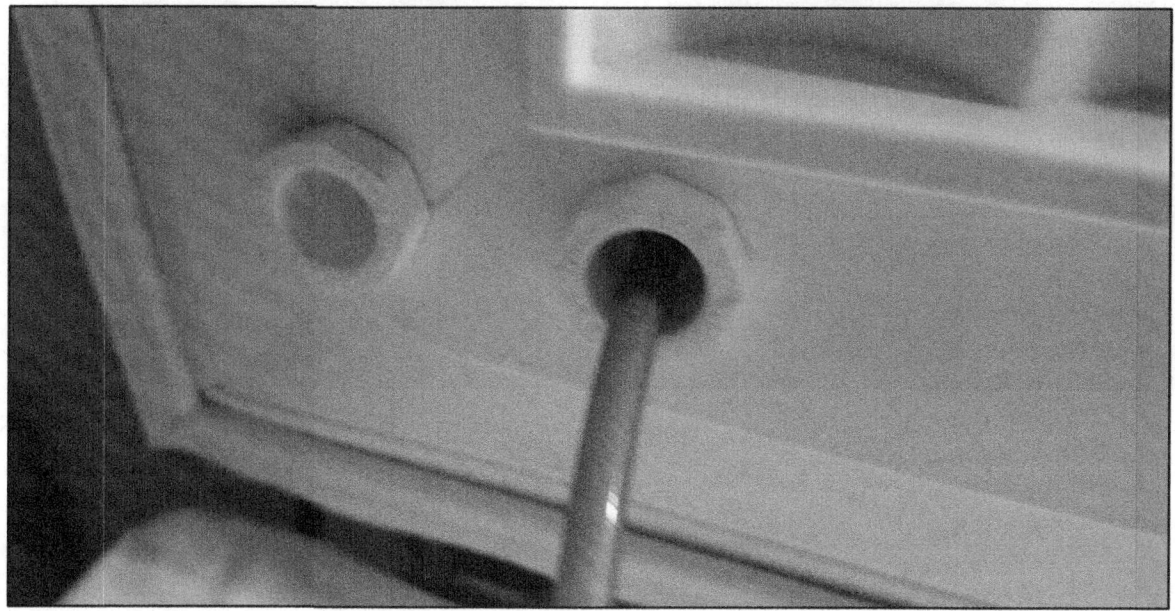

PVC plug inside the lid

CABLE MANAGEMENT

Use twist ties, wire ties, or Velcro straps to keep your cables neat and tidy.

Put one loop in your wires, cables, and tubes outside of the chest freezer. The loop is between the equipment/power and the water. If water splashes or condensation forms on the tubes or wires, it drips to the ground instead of somewhere it could cause damage.

I use a magnet with a small carabiner to keep my wires in place. Magnets are also a handy place to store the key.

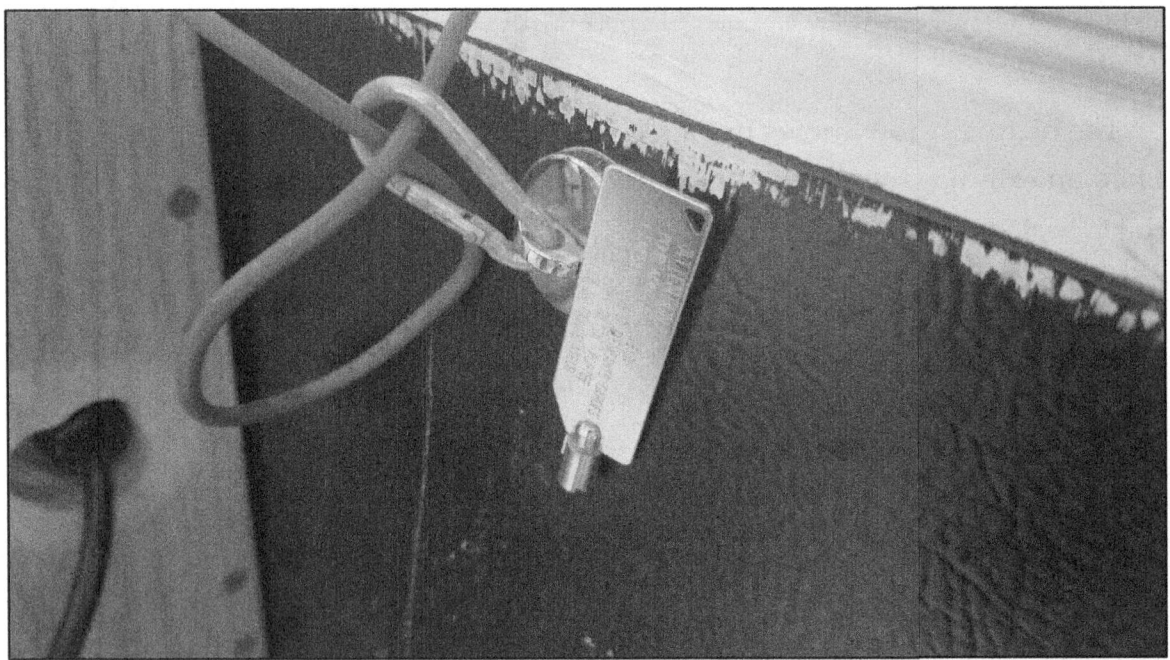

Magnet key & wire holder

EXAMPLE SETUP DIAGRAM

The below diagram shows a chest freezer connected with the following equipment:

- Submersible pump/filter

- Temperature controller

- Ozone generator

- GFCI with 3 outlets

- Timer

- Two heavy-duty extension cords (one long, one short)

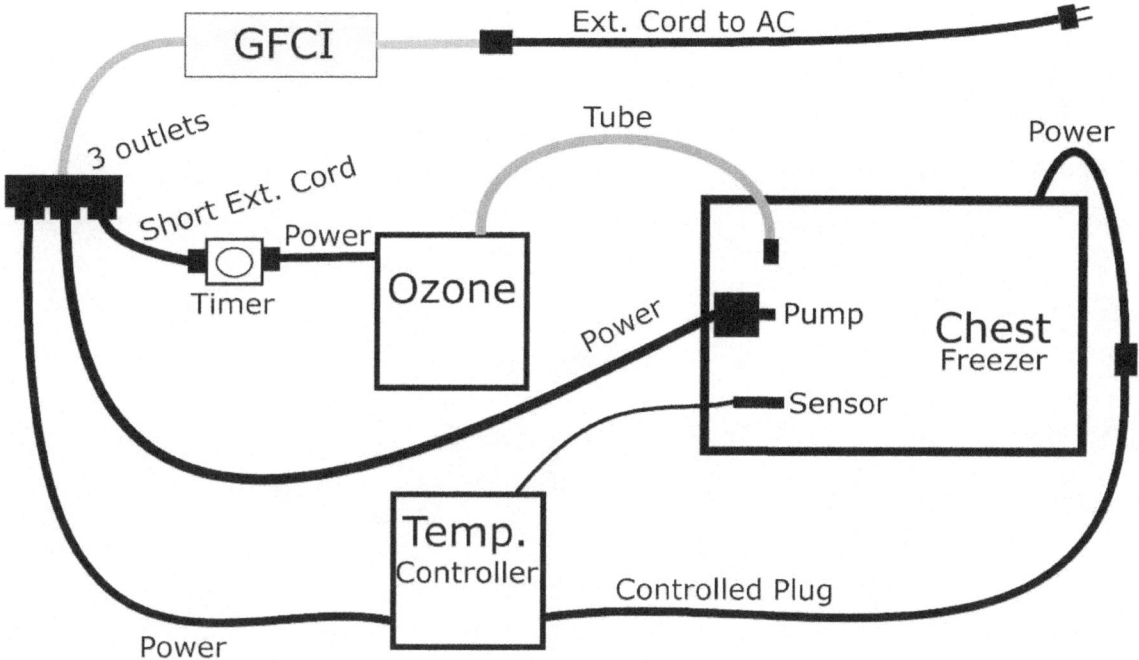

Connection diagram

" *Man can learn nothing except*
by going from the known to the unknown. "

Claude Bernar

Chapter 9: Introduction to Water Sanitation

Since the dawn of civilization, societies have known the importance of clean water. Because proper water sanitation is essential, three separate chapters are devoted to this topic.

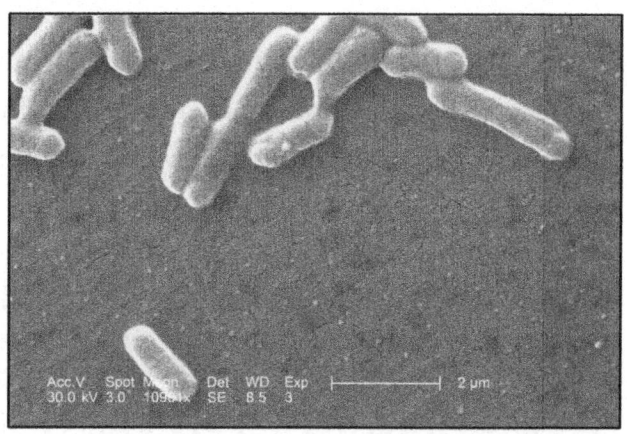

An E. coli colony seen through an electron microscope

Putting your body into unclean water can have consequences that range from inconvenient to life-threatening. The World Health Organization estimates that 3.575 million people die each year from water-related diseases. Most of these deaths come from drinking contaminated water, but the underlying message is relevant. If you want to stay safe and healthy, you need to keep your water clean.

Health problems can arise from contaminated water touching your skin, breathing vapor, or drops splashing into your nose, eyes, or mouth. Microorganisms, chemicals, or other contaminants in your water can result in these symptoms:

- Skin rash
- Itching
- Dry skin
- Diarrhea
- Stomach ache
- Ear and eye infections

- Nausea
- Vomiting
- Flu symptoms
- Pneumonia
- Death

THE MYTH OF CLEAN COLD WATER

Some cold-plungers assert that bacteria cannot live in cold water and therefore no extra steps for sanitation are necessary. It takes only a little bit of research to discover that bacteria can remain alive even when frozen for long periods.

For example, while E. coli needs a temperature range of 39-113°F (4- 45°C) to grow, it can survive refrigeration and freezing. It takes only 5 - 10 cells of viable E. coli to make you sick. Just think about how much that bacteria, floating in cold water, would love to find your warm skin!

This guide is not intended to provide in-depth knowledge of pathogens. Suffice to say, cold temperatures alone do not make your water safe to use.

 # AN OUNCE OF PREVENTION

The first step in keeping your water clean is to prevent or reduce the amount of stuff that gets in it. Here are a few tips:

1. Pre-Rinse or Shower
Take a shower, or at least rinse off immediately before you get in the water.
Do this every time.

2. Wear a swimsuit
A swimsuit helps reduce the amount of fecal matter that can get into the water.

3. Wear Shoes to Your Cold Plunge
Wear house shoes, sandals, or flip flops when walking to your chest freezer.
Remove your shoes before getting in.

4. Wipe Your Feet
Wipe your feet right before you get in. Have a mat in front of your chest freezer.

5. Wear a swim cap
A swim cap can reduce the amount of hair that can get into your chest freezer.

DRAIN & REFILL

If you prefer to keep things simple, all you need to do is drain your water as needed. How often depends on several variables. Every 3 – 7 days is a reasonable amount of time to start.

Pay attention to your water. If it is cloudy or smells funny, do not get in!

There are downsides to the drain and refill method:

1. It must be done frequently.

2. Each time you refill, it may take several days to chill your water to your desired temperature, resulting in lost training days.

3. Not all bacteria make your water cloudy or cause an odor.

Set up a strict schedule and stick to it.

Partial Draining

Some people report draining some of their water on a regular schedule. Their main reason being that it takes less time to cool down to the target temperature. However, this is not recommended. If bacteria are in your water, all of that water needs to be replaced in order to avoid risk.

THREE ESSENTIALS

Clear, clean water is a balance of three things:

1. Circulation

2. Filtration, and

3. Sanitation

Circulation moves the water and is necessary for filtration and sanitation methods to work effectively. *Filtration* removes large particulates such as oil, hair and skin flakes. *Sanitation* prevents growth of pathogens and bacteria. These three concepts will be discussed in detail over the next two chapters.

We can learn a lot about water sanitation from swimming pool and hot tub owners. Most of them spend significant time and money testing and keeping their water clean. Standard tests for pool and hot tub water include alkalinity, pH, hardness, and chlorine levels. Common problems include odors, water turning a weird color, cloudy water, scale, and algae build up.

A cold plunge is different than a hot tub or swimming pool; however, if you plan to sit in water for your health, it is vital to keep that water clean.

Some people don't want to think about this, but here is a list of a few things that can end up in your water:

- Dirt
- Skin flakes
- Oils from your body
- Sweat
- Residue from deodorant, soap, shampoo, and perfume

- Pieces of hair
- Insects
- Bacteria
- Microorganisms
- Algae
- Fecal matter, yes poop.

Trust me- you don't want to soak in that stew, much less dunk your head! Clean water is critical, and ignorance is not bliss!

Notes

_____

_____

_____

_____

_____

_____

_____

_____

_____

_____

_____

_____

_____

_____

_____

_____

" *Every success story is a tale of* "
constant adaption, revision and change.

Richard Branson

Chapter 10:
Chemicals & Additives

The many products available for water sanitation can be used alone or in combination with the devices discussed in Chapter 11. This chapter will explore a few products that can be used to sanitize your water.

CHLORINE, BROMINE, & ACIDS, OH MY!

DO NOT add spa chemicals to your cold plunge water unless you:

- have a pump and filter, and

- use the appropriate water tests!

Traditional methods of keeping the water clean in pools and hot tubs can be time-consuming, complicated, and expensive. If you don't believe me, just read through a few forums where pool and hot tub owners endlessly discuss the chlorine, bromine, neutralizers, levelers, balancers, pH increasers and decreasers, and shock treatments and when and how to use them and stop using them.

> **CAUTION**
>
> Chlorine will deteriorate aluminum. Do not use chlorine if you have a chest freezer with bare metal floors and walls.

Complaints about traditional pool chemicals include:

- Expense

- Time required

- Chemical odor

- Burning eyes

- Dry skin

- Coughing from fumes

- Bleached swimsuits

- Difficulty of use

- Long-term effect on health

Because of these reasons, unless you are already a pool or hot tub owner, have the chemicals and testing equipment available, and do not mind the extra time, I do not recommend going this route.

I did enough research to make this a definite "No" for myself. If you want to hear from someone who advocates pool chemicals, talk to your local pool equipment dealer, or read through the thousands of posts in dozens of different forums from people who are gung-ho about chlorine and other chemicals.

■ Simple Chlorine Option

Using a small floating chemical dispenser simplifies the use of chlorine. Test your water to maintain proper chlorine levels. See Chapter 15 for more information about maintenance.

As long as the chlorine level is correct, your water will be sanitized. If your water is too far off on any other tests, just drain and replace it.

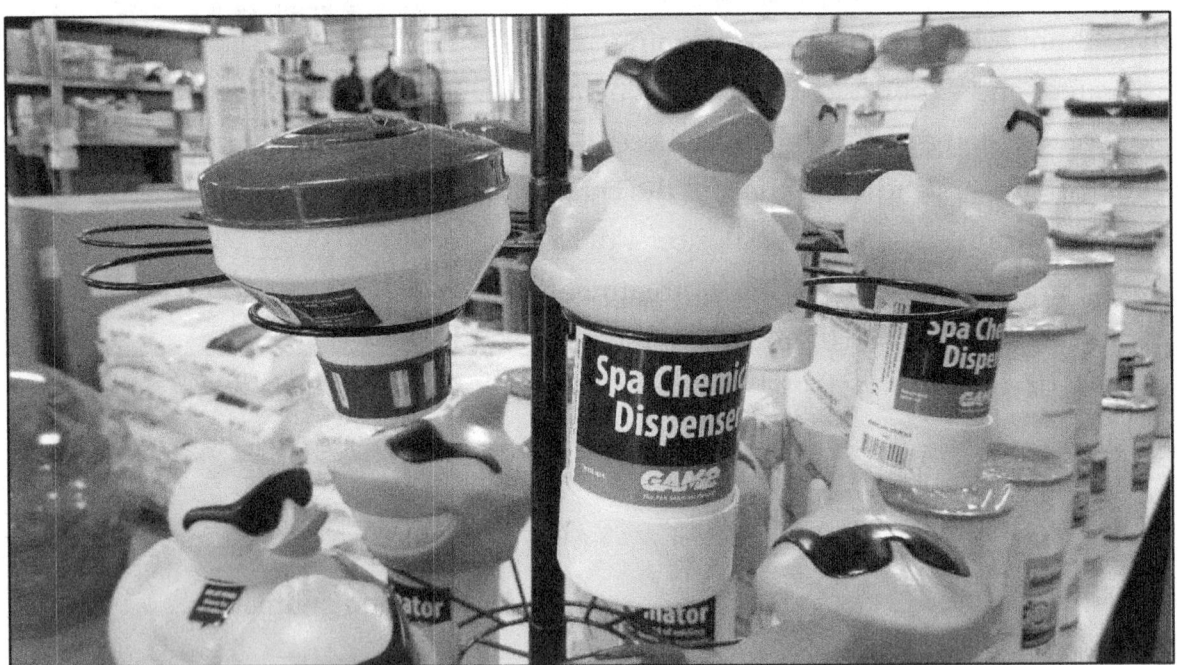

Chemical dispensers

If you do not have problems with chlorine or bromine, this is an easy way to go. The floating dispenser can be found at pool/hot tub supply stores for around $15. A 10 lb. (4.5 kg) bag of chlorine tablets costs about $50. A 1.5 lb. (.68 kg) container of bromine tables costs around $56.

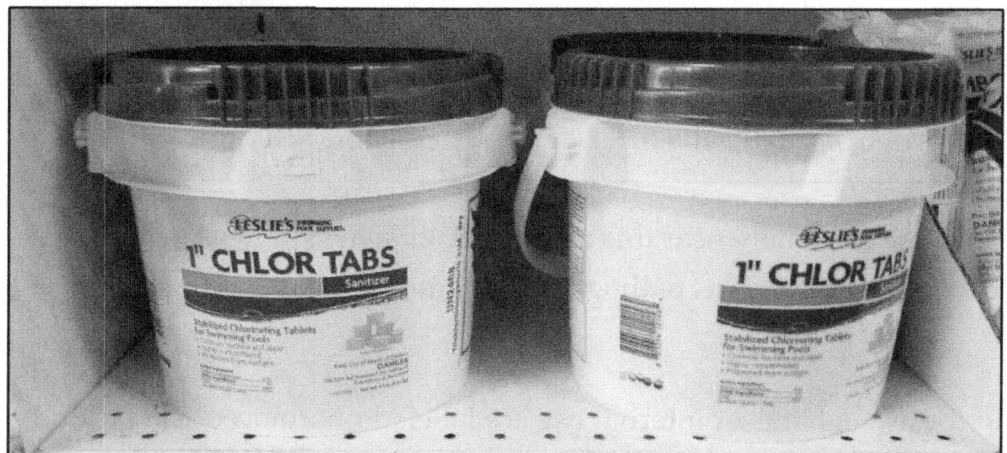

Chlorine tablets

 ## EPSOM SALTS

Epson salts have several benefits. They sanitize your water, lower the freezing point, and make your skin feel soft. However, you do need to use enough for them to make a difference- especially when it comes to sanitation.

> **CAUTION**
> Never mix Epsom salts with chlorine!

The formulas I found said a 10% salt solution would kill most bacteria that are harmful to humans. It did not specify if that was by weight or by volume. If we assume by weight, the approximate amounts are listed below for a few standard chest freezer sizes.

Here are a few notes:

- Weight of water: 8.4 lbs. (3.8 kg) per gallon

- Interior dimensions are used

- Waterline depth is 6 inches (15 cm) below the top of the wall

- The volumes account for the area displaced by the compressor cover

Volume of Chest Freezer	Volume of Water	Amount of Salt
7-cu. ft. / 198 L	39 gal. / 148 L	33 lbs. / 15 kg
15-cu. ft. / 424 L	75 gal. / 284 L	63 lbs. / 29 kg
21-cu. ft. / 594 L	108 gal. / 409 L	91 lbs. / 42 kg
25-cu. ft. / 708 L	179 gal. / 678 L	150 lbs. / 68 kg

Most people do not use anywhere near this amount of Epsom salt. Researching the amount of salt needed to kill various pathogens is behind the scope of this guide book.

Epsom salts sold for use in baths or internal use are labeled pharmaceutical or food grade. A 50 lb. (23 kg) bag of food-grade Epsom salt costs about $50.

Technical/Agricultural/Industrial grade Epsom salt is typically used on farms. The quality of the salt itself is essentially the same as food grade; however, it may contain impurities or heavy metals which could cause problems with water quality or leave residue.

I experienced this when I bought very cheap salts that I believe were incorrectly labeled as "food grade." Within one day, I had yellowish gunk on the walls of my chest freezer. A 50 lb. (23 kg) bag of technical grade Epsom salts runs about $20.

Technical grade is less expensive, and the impurities may not be a big deal; however, it's a good idea to invest the extra money for quality food grade Epsom salt from a reputable company.

It's up to you which one you use. However, as a point of reference, companies that sell float tanks (isolation tanks) recommend food-grade salts.

If you use Epsom or other salts, it is a good idea to rinse off afterward.

OTHER SALTS

You can buy Dead Sea and other mineral salts if you want more of a spa-type experience. However, they can be expensive.

Other formulations of salt are available, but because of limited information about their use or effectiveness, they are not included here.

The Downside of Salts

There are two main concerns with using salts in your cold plunge.

First, the salt may cause rust. Wipe up any water that has splashed or dripped.

The second concern is that the amount of salt needed to sanitize your water will make you more buoyant. You may not be able to easily get your shoulders underwater unless you hold the sides of the walls. Some people say that the best results from cold water immersion come when your body is completely relaxed in the water, so this may not be an ideal solution. You could use a weight (like a diver's weight belt), but this would add one more step to your routine.

HYDROGEN PEROXIDE

I have no personal experience using H2O2 as a water sanitizer, although I have used it for other purposes. Others report being very happy using H2O2 in their hot tubs and cold plunges.

> **CAUTION**
>
> Only use H2O2 if your water comes from a chlorinated municipal supply. If your water comes directly from a well, lake, or another natural source, do not use H2O2.

Here are a few tips about using H2O2:

1. Food grade (35%)

"Food Grade" means that it is safe to be used with food and contains no toxins. In the US, the Food and Drug Administration (FDA) has standards that must be met for a product to be labelled "food grade."

Keep in mind that just because something is labeled "food grade" does not mean that it is food grade. Buy from a reputable source.

Food Grade H2O2 comes in two concentrations: 35% and 50%.
Only the 35% concentration may be sold to the public.

8% and 12% H2O2 is not food grade.

It is best to purchase H2O2 that has
been certified food grade. While I do not
specifically endorse this website, the
link below has excellent info to help you
start your research:

> **FUN TRIVIA**
> H2O2 has a range of uses, depending on its concentration. Concentrations higher than 91% are used as rocket propellant... not available in pharmacies.

www.purehealthdiscounts.com

2. Beware of Technical Grade

I feel disheartened when people go through the effort to set up a cold plunge for
their health, and then cut corners on sanitizing to save a few dollars, thereby putting
their health at risk. Technical Grade H2O2 is cheaper than Food Grade, but it is not
recommended.

Manufacturing H2O2 is a complex
process. When used for industrial
purposes, the main goal is to make it as
cheaply as possible. Because of this,
heavy metals and chemicals are used as
stabilizers and can be bad for your
health if exposed to your skin or
ingested. Food grade H2O2 cannot be made at home.

> **COMPATIBILITY**
> Chest freezers with painted and unpainted interiors as well as pond and pool liners are all compatible with H2O2 levels needed to sanitize your water.

As a side note, if a website offers "organic" H2O2, be aware that there is no such
thing. H2O2 is a chemical, and neither water nor oxygen is "organic." Find
somewhere else to shop.

You will most likely not be able to find 35% food grade H2O2 at a local supplier and
will need to order it online.

Search online to find suppliers in your country or region. Shop around because
availability and prices can vary.

3. Safety
Use gloves when handling H2O2. It can damage your skin and eyes, and it bleaches clothing. It is corrosive and can be fatal if swallowed. Keep it away from children and pets. Always use child-proof caps. Use protective eye-wear.

"Gentlemen, don your goggles."
David Addison, Moonlighting

4. Initial Shock
An initial high amount of H2O2 helps prepare your water before your first use. You can shock the water after you fill it so that it will be ready to use when chilled.

Use eight ounces per 250 gallons (250 ml per 1,000 liters) of water. For example, if you have a cold plunge with 100 gallons (379 liters) of water, use 3.2 oz. (95 ml) of H2O2.

Use a glass measuring cup since glass is non-reactive to H2O2. Do not use metal measuring cups because they may react to the H2O2.

Let the water stand for one day before you get in. If you have a pump/filter (which I recommend!), let it run during this time. Check the filter after one day and clean or replace it if needed.

5. Testing your water
To ensure that your water is clean, use H2O2 test strips. They can be ordered from suppliers who sell H2O2 for spa and pool use. The recommended range is 30 - 100 ppm. Test your water at least once per week.

6. Maintenance
When the H2O2 levels drop below 40-50 ppm, add 8 oz. per 500 gallons (250 ml per 2,000 L) of water. This amounts to 1.6 oz. (47 ml) for 100 gallons (379 L).

Keep H2O2 levels below 100 ppm. Anything above 200 ppm can cause skin irritation.

7. H2O2 and Ozone

Pool and spa experts say that H2O2 is supposed to be used with an ozone generator or UV sterilizer; however, some people report that their water is clean without the additional equipment. You'll need to experiment to find what works best.

8. Pump/filter

It's a good idea to have a pump/filter because it ensures the H2O2 mixes with all of your water. We will discuss pumps in the next chapter.

9. Storage

H2O2 should be stored in a cool dark place away from other chemicals and any heat sources.

■ Alternatives to Pure Hydrogen Peroxide

Several people have reported good results with the products "Tank Safe" and "Ozone Clear." These products are meant to be used in hot tubs with ozone generators, not by themselves. They are mentioned here as a resource for you to consider, not as an endorsement of the product. There may be others. Search online or check with spa supply stores.

COLLOIDAL SILVER

Some hot tub and cold plunge users have recommended Colloidal Silver or colloidal silver generators for keeping their water clean. Out of the alternative methods available, this is probably the least discussed, although the folks who recommend it seem to be raving fans.

If purchased as a ready-made additive, colloidal silver can be expensive. People who use it for water sanitation usually purchase a colloidal silver generator.

I only did a bit of research on this product. At this point, I would consider it viable for our purpose, but untested.

ESSENTIAL OILS

Some cold plungers recommend tea tree oil as a non-toxic way to keep your water clean. I found many articles about using tea tree oil as a cleaner and disinfectant, but none for water sanitation. Essential oils can be used along with Epsom salts.

However, I did find information about using other essential oils in hot tubs instead of the traditional chlorine / bromine.

The bottom line is that it seems like no single essential oil by itself will take care of everything, but combining several together seems to work.

Which oils to use?

Eucalyptus, peppermint, lavender, cinnamon, and tea tree oil have anti-bacterial and anti-fungal properties.

Only pure essential oils should be used. Avoid low-quality brands that have other ingredients.

If you use any citrus essential oils, you should wait at least 24 hours before getting in the water because it might cause photo sensitivity.

How much to use?

One article I found said to use 3 drops of oil per person capacity of your hot tub. For a cold plunge smaller than 15 cu. ft. (400 L) that would be 3 drops of each oil. For larger chest freezers, 6 drops would work.

Another hot tub user said they use 10 drops of geranium oil and a cap full of Thieves oil once every two weeks- but that is for a large hot tub used only once per week.

Thieves is a specific product from Young Living oil, but you can find formulas online on how to make your own. One caution about Thieves is that it contains citrus oils, which can cause photo sensitivity in some people.

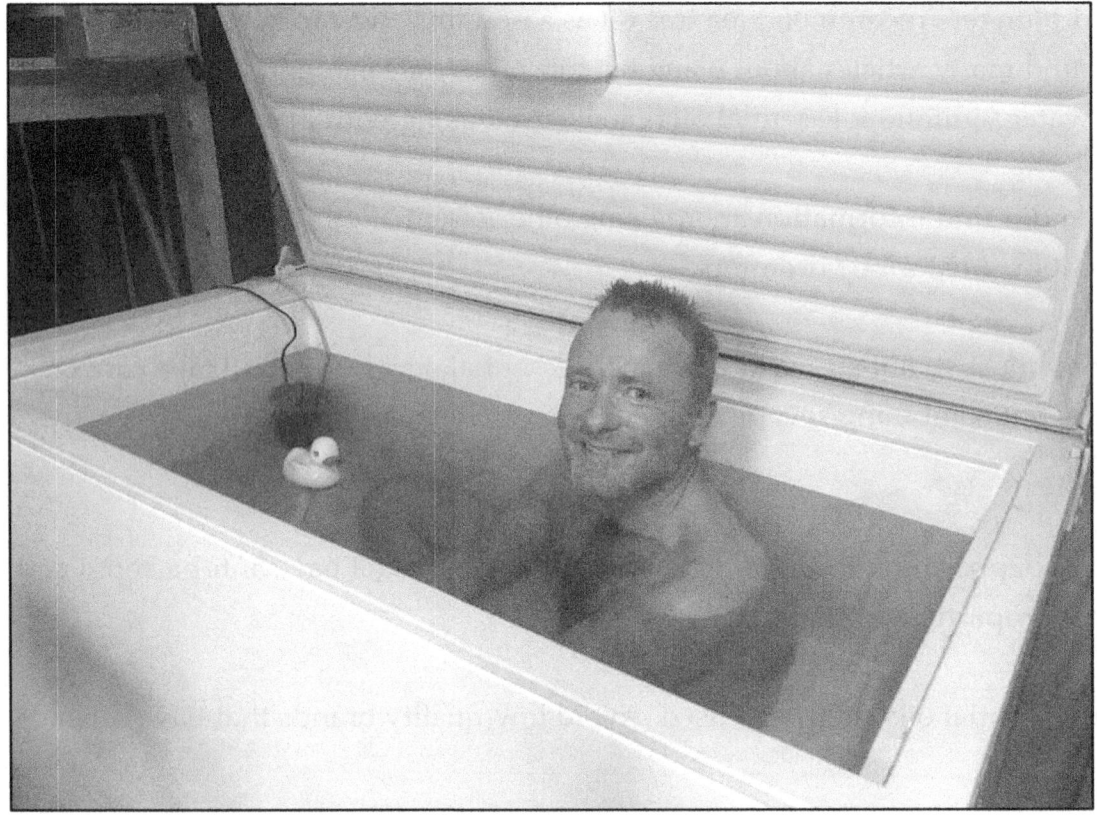

Jurgen H., Melbourne, Australia

Size: 500 L

Seams: Sealed with Selly's Wet Area Silicone

Water Sanitation: internal fish tank filter, wipe feet before entering

Water Temperature: Ranges from 0 ° - 1° C

Temperature Control: timer run 2-3 hours each night.

Training Protocol: Does 2-3 sessions between sauna and pool; ends in the freezer

Future Plans: Add ozone generator

Notes

_____

_____

_____

_____

_____

_____

_____

_____

_____

_____

_____

_____

_____

_____

_____

_____

_____

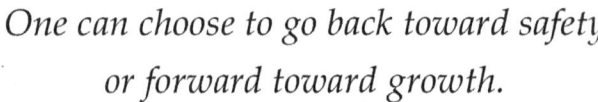

*One can choose to go back toward safety
or forward toward growth.*

*Growth must be chosen again and again;
fear must be overcome again and again.*

Abraham Maslow

Chapter 11: Water Sanitation Technology

In this chapter you'll learn about devices that can be used for water sanitation. Before we start, I'll mention two products to avoid.

Ionizers and colloidal silver generators *might* work, although they tend to be expensive. I'm not comfortable recommending these devices until we do more research and have positive long-term results. One known issue with ionizers is that they do not kill or neutralize nearly the same number of microbes or organic and inorganic materials as ozone.

There are three devices to consider for water sanitation:

1. Pump/filter

2. Ozone generator

3. UV Light

PUMP / FILTER

A mechanical pump/filter is one of the very first things I would recommend to upgrade your setup. Not only will the pump reduce or prevent ice build-up, but the filter helps keep your water free of sediment.

I have installed two external and two internal pumps and learned valuable lessons from each.

External Pumps

My first external pump was a 300 gallon (1,136 L) per minute aquarium canister filter. While the pump and filter worked well, my water still got cloudy after a few days of use. This was not a failure of the pump, but a lack of sanitation!

I added a spa-grade ozone generator, but unfortunately, the aquarium filter did not supply the correct pressure to make it work. That is when I decided to install an external hot-tub grade pump, filter, and ozone generator with a bunch of plumbing. I thought this would solve my problems. It was a tremendous amount of work, and although the result *looked* awesome, there were problems.

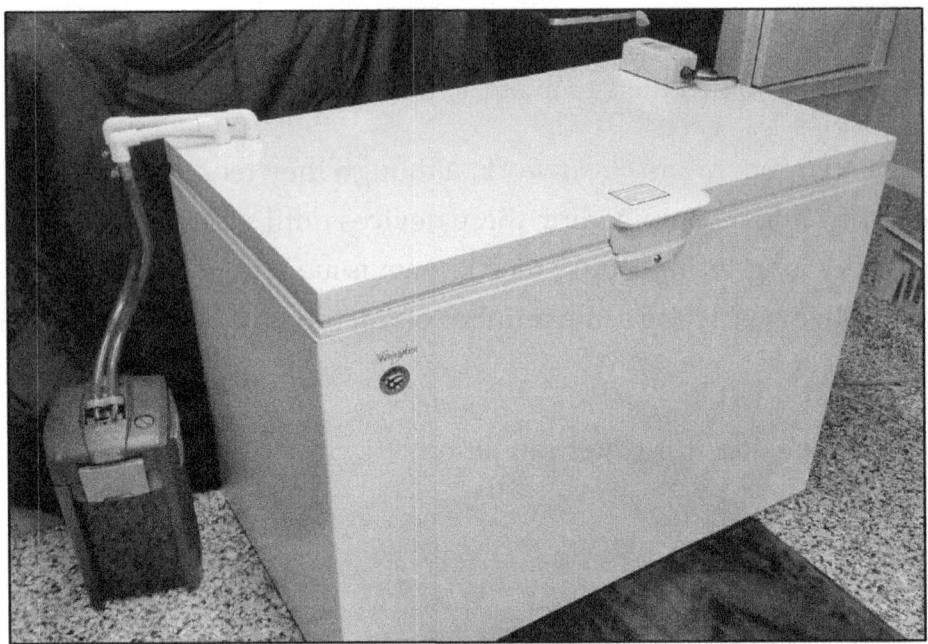

External aquarium canister pump/filter

Three critical issues with an external pump/filter are:

1. Getting the tubes/plumbing into and out of the chest freezer (drilling holes)

2. Condensation on the equipment and plumbing, and

3. Heat gain into your system prevents the water from getting cold enough.

I solved the first problem with varying levels of complexity, drilling holes in the lid for my aquarium filter, and eventually through the floor of the freezer to install the intake and return plumbing for the hot tub equipment. This, in turn, required a platform to elevate the chest freezer. I ended up building a great-looking deck but soon discovered this setup did not give me the cold water that I wanted.

The biggest problem with external plumbing is the condensation and heat gain. The difference in temperature made the tubes/plumbing sweat. While this was not as big of a deal with the smaller canister filter which only had a few feet of tubes, on the spa set up, I had more than 14 feet of pipes and valves as well as the pump and filter.

All of this made a mess on my porch, but worse, prevented my water from getting any colder than 48° F (8.8° C).

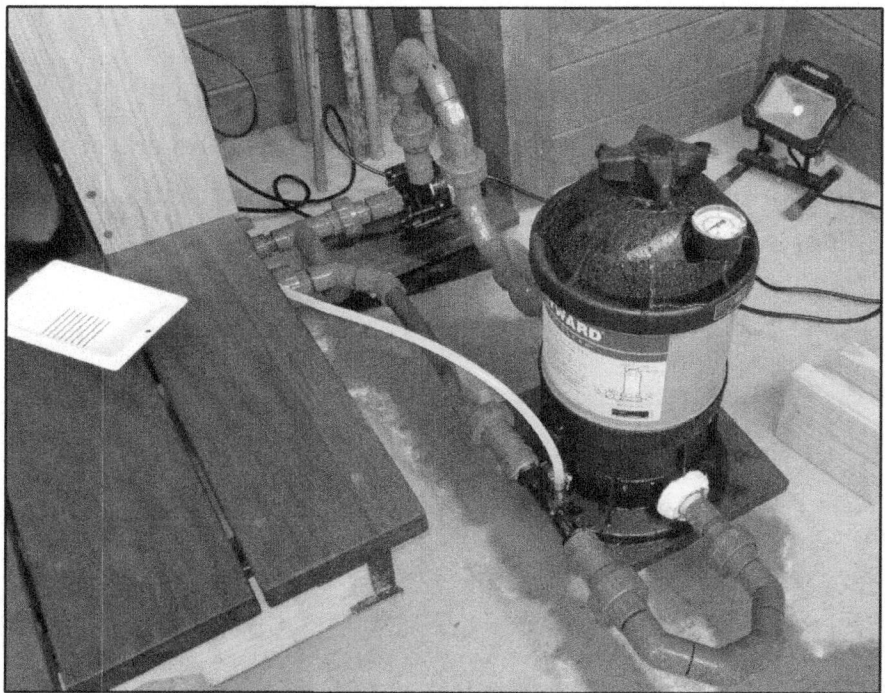

External hot-tub pump, filter, and plumbing

I started researching insulation and how to reduce the amount of condensation/heat gain. At one point I talked with an industrial engineer who said that the temperatures in Central Texas would require closed-cell foam insulation of at least 2" in diameter around all of the pipe and the equipment.

The cost was several hundred dollars for the materials, but there was no way of knowing it could be correctly installed around the pump, filter, and valves, or sealed correctly. I felt nervous about the risk of money and time, with no guarantee that it would work.

I looked into buying a sizeable walk-in freezer that would hold the entire setup and found out they are crazy expensive, and have special electrical requirements that standard home outlets would not provide. I wanted to press on, but remembered the "sunk cost" fallacy (see the note at the end of the chapter), and finally cut my losses.

With a heavy heart, I disassembled the entire setup and threw all of the plumbing and filters into a dumpster.

Internal Pumps

Internal submersible pumps are my current "best practice" recommendation. They are inexpensive, simple to use, and easy to maintain.

My first submersible aquarium pump was specified to handle 80 GPH (300L PH), which is the amount of water in my 15-cu. ft. (424 L) chest freezer. However, there were two issues. First, it did not prevent ice from forming, and second, without a filter, there was still sediment in my water.

Optimal Flow Rate

When sizing an internal pump, find one that has a flow rate of at least 2-3 times the volume of water. So, for example, if you have 80 gallons (300 L), it would be best to purchase a pump that has a flow rate of 160 or 240 gallons per hour (600 – 900 L/H).

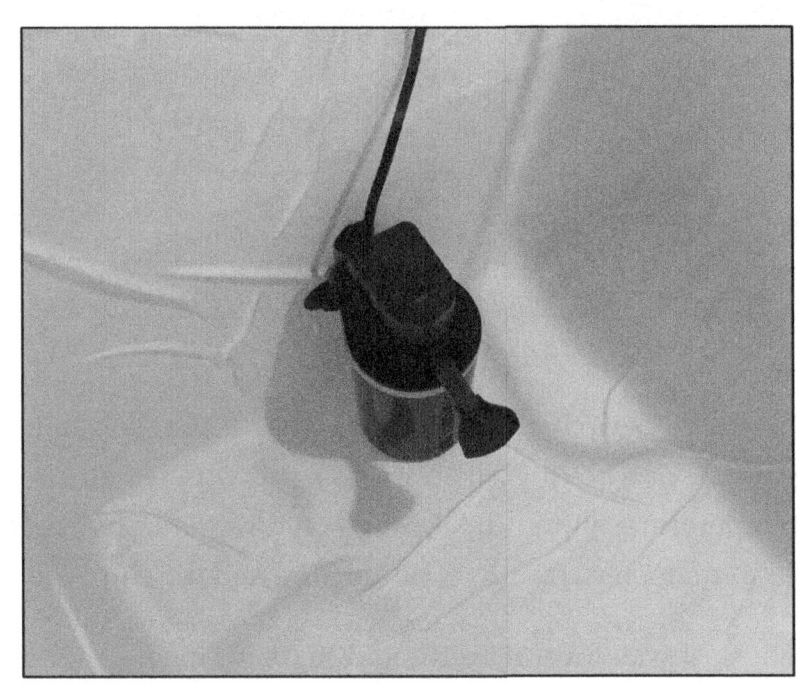

MarineLand submersible pump

The second submersible aquarium pump I found was from MarineLand. It was rated for 290 gallons per hour (1,198 L/H) and had a built-in filter. After being in use for more than 18 months now, it has performed very well. Not only does the circulation completely prevent ice from building up (at 36° F/2.2° C), the filter catches loose hair and other particles.

Filters

The MarineLand pump comes with two types of filters. One is a carbon bio-filter, and the other is a standard sediment filter, which they call the "polishing filter." Use the polishing filter. Be sure to place the rubber gasket into the canister or debris can escape the filter.

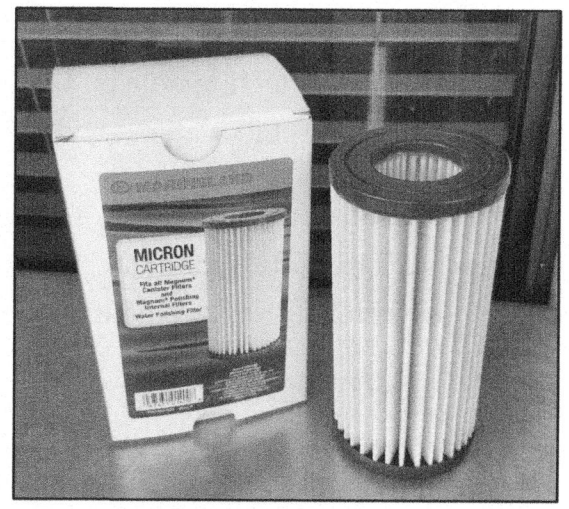
MarineLand replacement polishing filter

I found it helpful to buy a spare filter, and swap them out when I clean it. You might need to change and clean your filter once per week. At a minimum, change and clean the filter at least once per month.

I use my filter along with an ozone generator, and my water has been clean and crystal clear for as long as five months. The only reason it was not in use longer than that was because I moved.

Buy an aquarium filter that is fully submersible. Some are designed to be attached to the edge of the aquarium wall and require an intake that is above the waterline. This does not work well in a chest freezer set up because of the thickness of the walls prevents the bracket from attaching, and the lid from closing.

The MarineLand Magnum Polishing Pump/Filter rated for 290 GPH (1,098 LPH) sells for around $50.

Others have reported good results using pond and fountain pumps and filters. I have a preference for aquarium filters because they are specifically designed not to kill fish. If they are safe for fish, they should be safe for people!

Some people put their pump on a timer; however, I don't recommend it. Aquarium, pond, and fountain pumps are meant to run continuously, and frequent starting and stopping can shorten the life of the motor.

Stuck Filters

A few people have reported the MarineLand filter swelling and getting stuck in the housing. After collecting data on the issue, it seems to be a manufacturer defect that is affected by the cold water.

Some solutions include: getting a replacement under warranty, filling it with warm water and letting it sit for a day, use salad/food tongs to remove the filter. Those who have received replacements have reported no issues.

OZONE GENERATORS

For people who are sensitive to chlorine or don't want to use chemicals, ozone is an excellent choice for sanitation. Ozone has been used to sanitize municipal drinking water since 1906. Ozone generators for hot tubs were introduced in the 1980s.

Ozone sanitizes and disinfects, and is many times stronger than bromine and chlorine. Ozone can kill 99% percent of all microbes (viruses and bacteria), as well as cysts, fungus, algae, and mold. Ozone oxidizes oils and other contaminants in the water. Oxidized particulates clump together, which is why you need to use a pump and filter to remove them from the water.

The only byproduct of using an ozone generator is oxygen. It does not damage the environment or

Ozone molecules, included because I think they look cool!

atmosphere. Ozone in the water will not irritate or dry out your skin.

There are two basic ways to generate ozone, Ultra Violet (UV) light and Corona Discharge (CD). The CD ozone produces higher amounts of ozone, and is typically recommended by high end spa companies.

The main disadvantage of the UV models is that the expensive UV lamps have low output and must be replaced frequently.

Do not run units while using your cold plunge because breathing ozone can damage your lungs. There is no need to worry about ozone building up in your chest freezer. It dissipates quickly.

■ Using Ozone with Other Products

Even with ozone, traditional hot-tub suppliers still recommended using standard chemicals and a backup sanitizer "just in case." Using ozone greatly reduces the amount of chemicals needed, however, a growing number of hot-tub owners report success using only ozone. The disadvantage with doing that is there is no way to test your water to ensure that it is sanitized.

Ozone is compatible with other water sanitation solutions, including standard pool chemicals (chlorine and bromine), H_2O_2, ionizers, salt, and UV light.

■ Maintenance Tips

While ozone sanitizes your water, it won't clean the walls or floor of your chest freezer. If your walls or floor feel slick or slimy, this is most likely because of algae growth. Wipe the walls with the soft side of a sponge. Your pump/filter will catch the sediment. If too much slime builds up on your walls or floor, drain the water and clean the tub.

■ Hot Tub Ozone Generators

In hot tubs, ozone is mixed with water by a device called a venturi injector. The downside is that the injector must be installed inline with external plumbing.

Unless you want to spend an additional $400 - $600 on the setup, external pumps are a huge hassle and do not work well.

Not only is there significant condensation with external plumbing, but the heat gain in the plumbing and components makes it difficult (or impossible) for your chest freezer to chill the water to your desired temperature.

■ The Stand-Alone Ozone Generator

The good news is that stand-alone ozone generators are available. A built-in pump pushes the ozone through a tube and into a diffuser stone which mixes it into the water. You must have a separate pump/filter for stand-alone ozone generators to work well. Without a pump circulating your water, it will not be sanitized.

■ Testing

While there is no easy way to test for pathogens in your water, there is an easy way to test ozone levels. Ozone test strips are available from a number of online retailers. If you have no issues with your water, you can probably get away with test just once per month. Test kits of 50 strips are available for about $20 on Amazon. Check the water while your ozone generator is running. Ozone meters are available, but cost hundreds or thousands of dollars.

There are three key things to look for to ensure that your ozone generator is working:

1. **Clear Water**
   If you water is not crystal clean, your ozone generator or check valve might need to be replaced.

2. **Odor**
   Ozone has a distinct pungent but fresh smell. You should notice it when you open the lid after the ozone generator has run. A funky smell is a sign that bacteria could be building up.

3. **Age**
   If your ozone generator is older than one to three years, it most likely needs to be replaced. Some ozone generators have replaceable parts. With others, the entire device needs to be replaced.

■ Maintenance

Once per year you should replace your check valve and ozone tubing.

JED Engineering

One company that makes this type of ozone generator is JED Engineering. You'll need to order it from a retailer. The specific model that I use and recommend is JED 203. It comes with the tube and bubbler stone. It plugs into a standard power outlet, but you need to specify what kind of plug you need when you order.

It can handle tanks up to 2,000 gallons (7,571 L), so it will definitely work on your chest freezer. If you live in the US, order the 120V model, and specify the "A Cord," which plugs into a standard outlet.

If you live in another country, order the 240V model and tell them to leave off the plug. You'll need to buy and attach a plug that fits the outlet where you live. These plugs are available at hardware stores. You might need a tool to strip the wires, along with a screwdriver to attach the bare wires to the plug.

Do NOT use travel adapters!

The JED 203 model comes with a 7' (2 meter) tube that is easy to work with. The built-in pump will send ozone through the diffuser stone under as much as 4 feet (1.2 meters) of water, allowing it to sit on the floor of your chest freezer. Since ozone bubbles upward, I believe it sanitizes more water when the diffuser stone sits on the floor.

The complete JED 203 package typically sells in the US for around $270. You can buy one from my website at https://chestfreezercoldplunge.com/. I ship globally.

The Corona Discharge assembly has a life expectancy of about 2 years, if the unit is run 24/7. The life expectancy will be much longer if you use a timer and run it less than 2-3 hours a day. I currently run mine for 30 minutes a day.

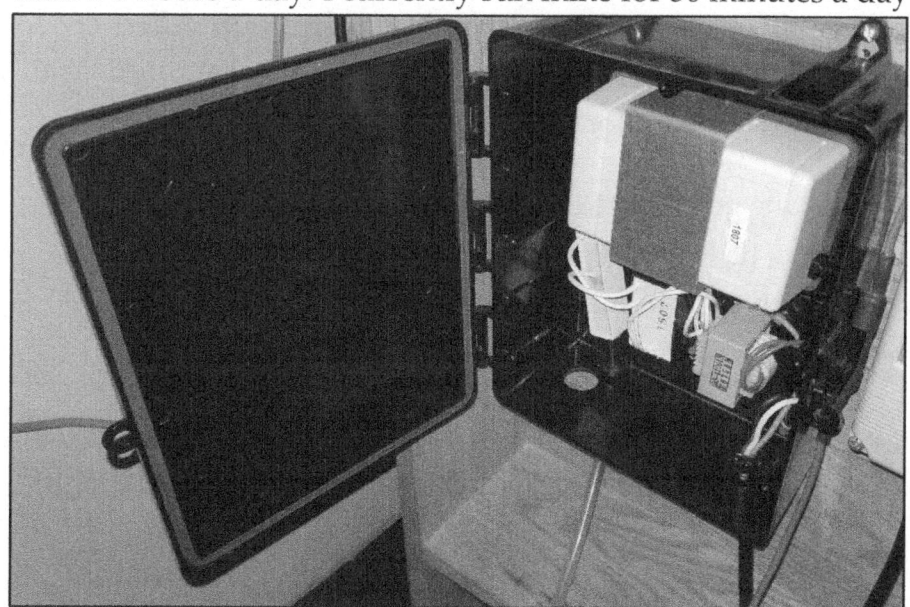

JED 203 ozone generator

A2Z Ozone

A2Z Ozone, Inc. makes ozone generators that have good reports from a growing number of people on our Facebook group. All of their products are available with voltage and plugs that work in the US, EU, UK, and AU.

While they have a full range of ozone generators for different purposes, they have two low priced models available: Aqua 6 for $78 and Aqua 8 for $134, both of which are designed for general home use.

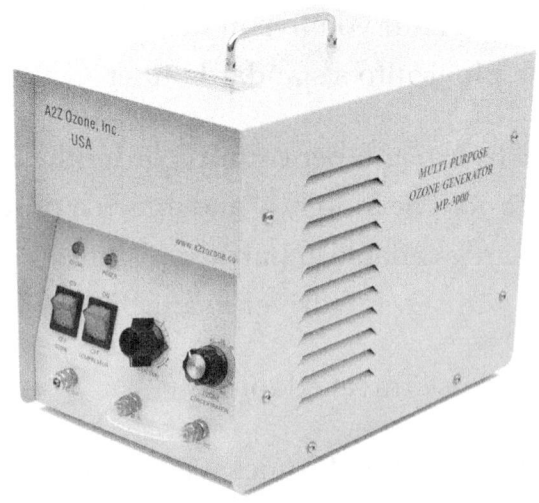

MP-3000 ozone generator

I mention these only because a lot of people buy them looking for a low-cost ozone generator, but these simply will not do the job.

A downside is that the Aqua-6 and 8 models only come with a 3' (1 meter) tube. Because of the smaller pumps in these units, longer tubes may not work well. A significant downside is that the diffuser stone on Aqua models should not be placed more than 4 inches (10 cm) under water. They are, after all, designed to be used in your kitchen. If you place the diffuser stone deeper than that, the pump will not push out as much ozone and you risk not having your water be fully sanitized. You also risk reducing the life of the pump motor.

They make more powerful ozone generators (with stand-alone pumps) that are designed for pool and spa use. The MP-1000 model is the one that will work, but you have to run it manually each time. The MP-3000 has a continuous run mode which, when used with an external timer, will give you what you need. It retails for $399.

Pleaser order from my link affiliate link us use the coupon code for a 12% discount:

https://tinyurl.com/A2ZMP3000

Coupon Code: CFCP12

UV LIGHTS

UV light will take care of 99.99% of microorganisms and is an FDA approved method to sanitize water. The main difference between ozone and UV is that while ozone kills microorganisms, UV alters the DNA or RNA so they cannot reproduce. Ozone will eliminate odors, while UV will not.

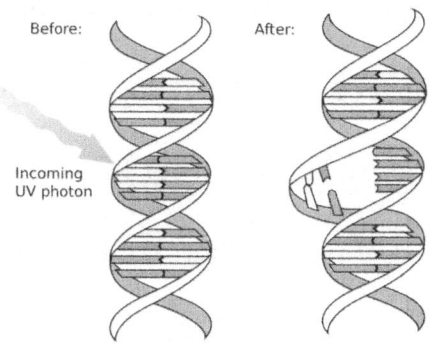

UV harms DNA

It must be used along with a pump/filter because UV won't work if the water is cloudy, and the microorganisms must be exposed directly to the UV light. Another issue is that when water is exposed to the UV light, it can raise the temperature several degrees.

As with ozone generators, UV systems used for pools and hot tubs are connected to the hot tub plumbing. The simple setup for your cold plunge is a submersible UV light with a built-in pump/filter.

However, there are several things to consider when choosing a UV product.

First, only specific UV light frequencies sanitize water. Without going into technical details, the one to use is UVC. Do not buy UVA or UVB bulbs.

Clarification and Sterilization

Next, it is important to know that UV light can either clarify or sterilize water, and there is a significant difference between these two actions.

Greenish water is a common problem for aquarium and pond owners. UV clarification will turn that green water clear, but it won't take care of the microbes in the water that can make you sick.

There are two levels of sterilization:

Level 1: Kills bacteria and some viruses

Level 2: Kills bacteria, most viruses, and parasites.

For our purpose, a level 1 is sufficient.

Most UV pump/filters sold on Amazon or eBay will only clarify your water.

There are a lot of technical details that explain the difference. If you are interested, check out this website for more information:

http://www.americanaquariumproducts.com

Their website has a wealth of information. Here are five of the many details they discuss:

1. Water must be clear for UV to work
2. The length of the UV lamp
3. How long the water takes to flow past the lamp
4. The assembly around the lamp
5. The flow pattern in the water

Another issue is that the effectiveness of UV sterilization depends on the water temperature. Colder water requires a longer exposure to UV light for proper sanitation.

The SunSUN AAP CUP-613, pictured below, is a good choice. Avoid the less expensive models.

The owner from A2Z said that for water temperatures of 32 - 57° F (0 – 13.9° C), two of these models would be needed, but that you would need to figure out how to slow down the flow rate on the output. He suggested putting some kind of barrier in front of the output. Never impede the input!

Two models will provide sterilization for 75 - 125 gallons (284 – 473 L) of water.

Any UV system that sells for less than $60 - $80 will typically be an inferior product that will not sanitize your water.

■ Using a UV Pump/Filter

Experts in the pool and spa industry say that UV is not a complete solution by itself. Small amounts of chlorine or food grade (35%) hydrogen peroxide can be added.

So far, those using UV without the added chemicals report good results, however, as mentioned in the previous section, there are many variables that need to be in place for UV to sterilize the water. Most people using UV are using inexpensive models, which will clarify the water, but not sanitize it. Their health is at risk!

Do not leave the UV light on 24/7. In fish aquariums, it only needs to run for 2 – 4 hours once every 3 – 4 days. I have not personally used a UV lamp, and do not yet have feedback from anyone else about their schedule. It's something you'll have to figure out.

Inspect the UV bulb and housing to make sure there are no cracks, and clean the built-in filter once every week or as needed.

The only maintenance required is to replace the lamp and sleeve once every 6 – 12 months.

Quality submersible UV lights with a pump/filter start at $85 and go up from there. Avoid cheap replacement bulbs.

■ External Aquarium UV Filters

External UV filters used for aquariums will typically provide adequate sanitation. However, they must be plumbed inline with an external pump and filter in order to work. Because of the issues of heat gain with an external pump/filter, I do not recommend this kind of setup unless you have serious DIY skills.

COMBINING OZONE & UV

There are differences in how ozone and UV work. If you use ozone, you really don't need to us UV. If you use UV, it is a good idea to add ozone, in which case you really wouldn't need UV.

If you choose to use both, a Corona Discharge (CD) ozone generator is needed.

Real World Benefits

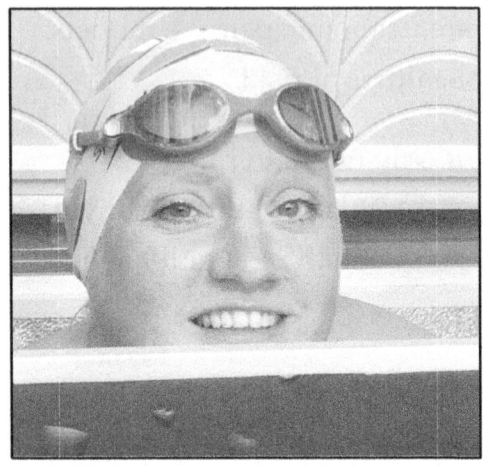

Catherine P. in her chest freezer training for an Antarctica swim

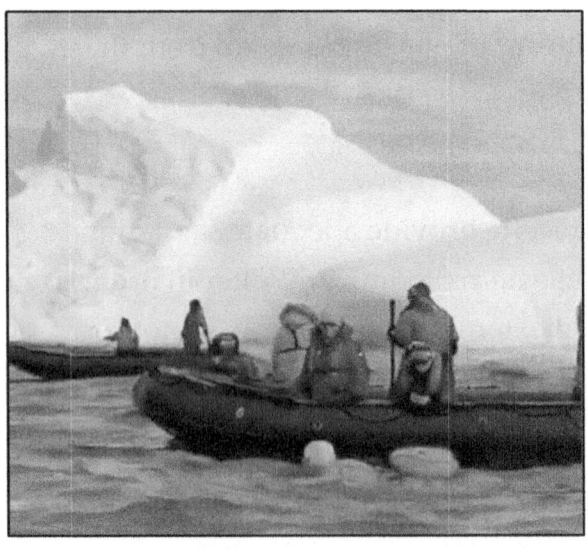

Catherine and her support team

UPDATE: On Feb. 22, 2020, Catherine became the first person in world history to swim an ice mile swim inside the polar Antarctic circle. The water temperature was 0° C (32° F).

NOTE: This requires special training. For most people, it is unnecessary to have your cold plunge water temperature set below 1.1° C (34° F).

■ Sunk Cost Fallacy

Members of our online group have asked questions about the meaning of the "sunk cost fallacy," so it is worth a brief tangent to go into more detail. This idea can be helpful not only in building a chest freezer, but in life.

Human nature influences us to keep doing things into which we have invested money and time. We like to think that we make rational decisions based on the future value our efforts or the things we own. However, our decisions are largely affected by our emotions.

The more money, time and focus we put into a project, the more emotionally attached we become, and the harder it is to stop.

Putting resources into something that is unlikely to give you a positive return is a huge waste. Unfortunately, this can happen in all areas of life, from our homes and cars, to our jobs, investments and relationships.

It also happens with chest freezers, and I'm the first one to stand up and say "Guilty!" For the money that I spent fixing mistakes in my chest freezer setups, I could have bought five or six new chest freezers and started over.

Either way, I learned from the mistakes. But repairing those mistakes to get the chest freezer back up to the baseline to try the next thing cost money and time- a lot of time. But I didn't want to throw away my chest freezer because I was emotionally invested!

Where is the line? It's up to you to decide, but here are a few thoughts.

If have a new chest freezer up and running and see some rust, it is worth it to redo your seals at that point.

If you buy a used chest freezer and have problems, it may be best to start over.

One of the main goals of this guide is to help prevent costly mistakes.

Here is a general guideline: if the cost to repair is more than half the price to replace it, then start over.

I encourage people to post about their mistakes and failed setups on our Facebook group. That is how we all learn, grow, and get better.

Real World Setup

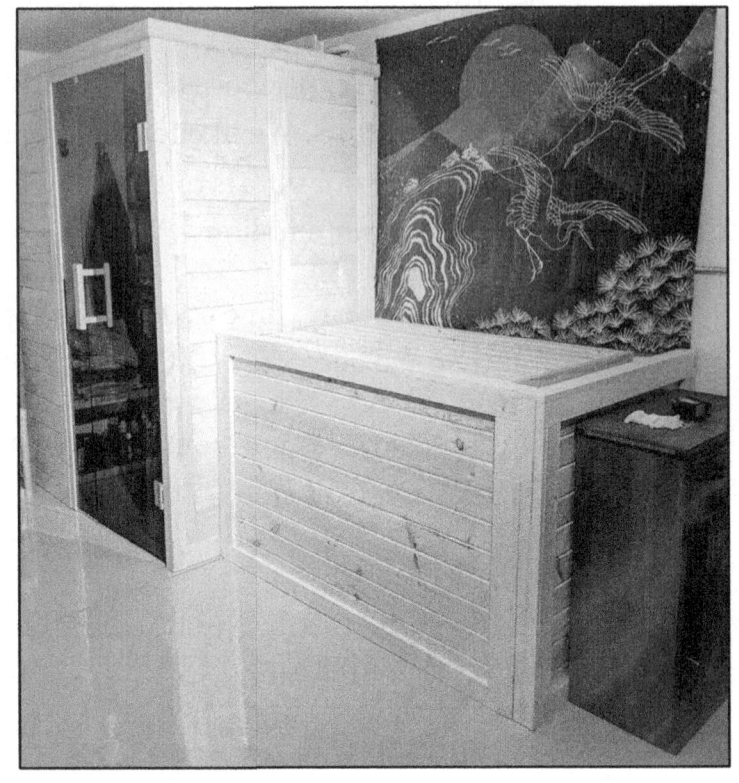

Chest Freezer:
Whirlpool model WZC3115DW01

Size: 500 L

Seams: Sealed with JB Water Weld

Support Underneath:
Anti fatigue mats from Harbor Freight, with holes cut out for the feet

Water Sanitation:
Mini adjustable floating dispenser for 1" chlorine tabs

Water Temperature:
Started at 58F (14.4C), planning to work their way down below the 40F (4.4C) range as they get adjusted

Temperature Control:
Inkbird ITC 308

Training Protocol:
Cycle through one or two times with the sauna, ending on cold unless they are under the weather or stressed in some other way like lack of sleep.

Exterior: Custom built cabinet from southern yellow pine, with 4" of space around outside walls of freezer for ventilation

Future Plans: build a step for easier access

Notes

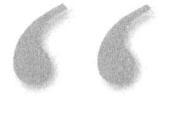 *The great solution to all human problems is individual inner transformation.*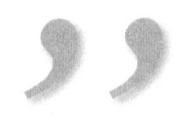

Vernon Howard

Chapter 12:
Examples of Chest Freezer Cold Plunge Systems

■ SAFETY

Water and electricity don't mix. Chest freezers are not designed or built to hold water. Aquarium pumps and other equipment are not meant to be used with people in the water. To keep yourself safe,

BEFORE YOU GET IN- UNPLUG EVERYTHING!

If the light comes on when you open the lid, your freezer is still plugged in.

Remember this: See the light? Unplug, alright!

Unplug it!

Anything else that is plugged in as part of your setup must also be unplugged. That includes pumps/filters, ozone generators, UV lights, and temperature controllers.

■ Do Not Try This at Home

There are a few setups that I do not recommend. Doing any of the following can shorten the life of your chest freezer or prevent your water from getting cold enough.

1. A chest freezer that has not been properly waterproofed/sealed.

2. Pumping water from a chest freezer into another tank.

3. External pumps or plumbing.

■ THE CAVEMAN

Cost: $150 - $300

You already know about filling bathtubs, trash bins, or stock tanks with ice. However, there is one other creative option that gets your chest freezer into the action.

This option works very well for those who prefer to spend 30 – 45 minutes in water between 50 - 57°F (10 - 13° C).

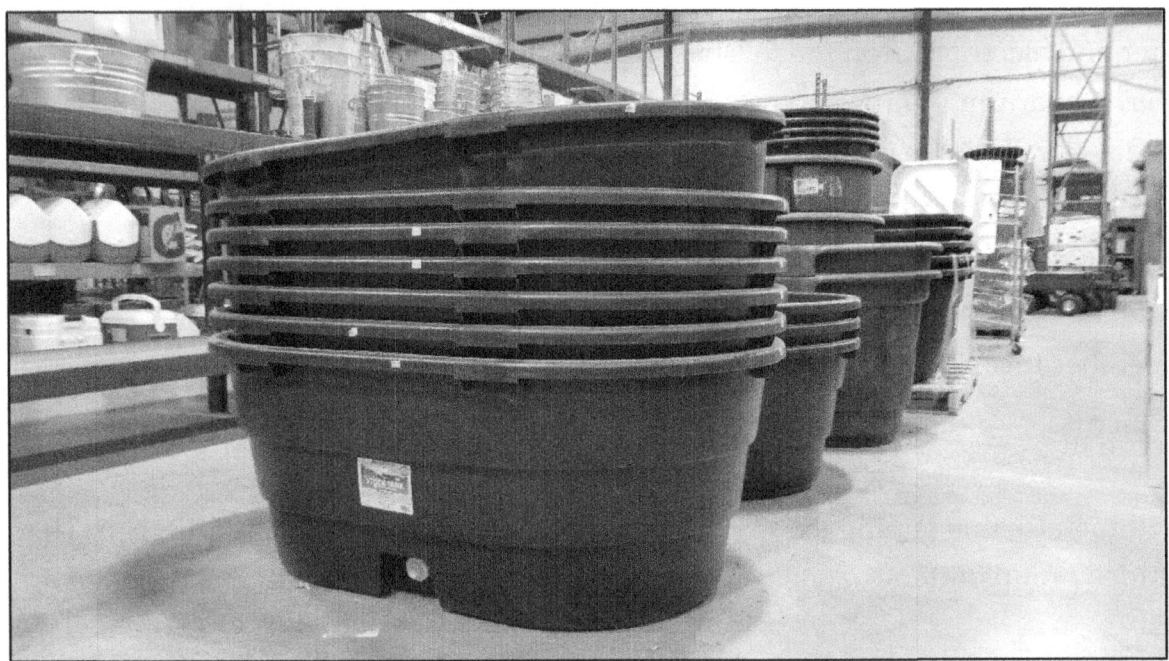

100-gallon (378 L) stock tanks

Fill a bunch of plastic bottles with water and put them in your chest freezer.

As soon as you have frozen water, put the containers into your bathtub or stock tank long enough to chill the water to your desired temperature. Put them back in your chest freezer when you finish, and enjoy the cold water.

This method requires a bit of work and extra time with each cold-water immersion; however, some people prefer a setup that requires no modifications to the chest freezer.

Because your chest freezer is being used as intended (to freeze foodstuffs), the warranty remains intact.

Materials

1. Used 8.7-cu. ft. (246 L) chest freezer

2. Your bathtub or a 100-gallon (378 L) stock tank

3. Thermometer

4. A bunch of plastic containers
    a. Approximate size: 1 gallon / 4 liters
    b. How many? See below.

Steps

1. Fill containers with water and place them in your chest freezer

2. Add water to your stock tank, leaving 6-8 inches from the top

3. When ready to do a cold immersion, place the containers of frozen water in your stock tank until your water has reached your desired temperature.

4. Remove the containers and put them back in your chest freezer. It may take 1 - 2 days for the water to completely freeze inside of the containers.

5. Enjoy your cold water.

When filling the containers with water, leave about an inch or two of air at the top to allow room for the water to expand as it freezes.

How many containers will you need? Several variables affect this, including the size of the containers and your starting and desired water temperature.

Appendix A shows the formula to figure out the amount of crushed ice needed to chill water. That calculation gets you close to the number of containers you need.

Example
If you have 80 gallons (300 L) of water at 80° F (26.7° C), it takes about 17 - 20 one-gallon (3.8 L) jugs to chill the water to 40° F.

What size of chest freezer do you need?

It depends on the size of your containers and how many you'll need to chill your water to your target temperature.

I found 1-gallon containers that measured 8" x 4" x 12" (20 cm x 10 cm x 30 cm).

An 8.7-cu. ft. (~221 L) chest freezer holds approximately 17 one-gallon containers without having to double stack. You could add another eight or ten jugs before it would be full.

A 15-cu. ft. (400 L) chest freezer would give you plenty of room. Having a larger chest freezer can be helpful if you decide to go for the full chest freezer cold plunge conversion.

Depending on your ambient temperature, it may take several days for the water in the containers to re-freeze.

Science Bonus: Add 1/2 to 1 lb. (226 to 453 g) of Epsom salts to each gallon container for quicker freezing.

*"What is it with you and the caveman thing?" she asked.
And why, oh why, do I like it so much?"*

Jill Shalvis, The Sweetest Thing

TEST DRIVE

Cost: $200 - $350

If you're not ready to commit to a full setup, this is an excellent way to test the waters. It is simple, easy, and inexpensive.

Other equipment can be added as you go.

Materials
1. Used chest freezer (15-cu. ft. / 424 L)

2. EPDM Pond liner

BASIC

Cost: $600 - $700

Materials
1. New Chest freezer (15-cu. ft. / 424 L)

2. JB Water Weld

3. Digital timer

4. Floating chemical dispenser & chlorine tablets

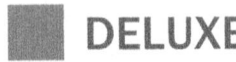

PLUNGE 2.0

Cost: $700 - $800

Materials

1. New chest freezer (15-cu. ft. / 424 L)

2. JB Water Weld

3. Temperature controller

4. Internal pump/filter

DELUXE

Cost: $900 - $1,200

Materials

1. New chest freezer (15-cu. ft. / 424 L)

2. JB Water Weld

3. Temperature controller

4. Internal pump / filter

5. JED 203 ozone generator

6. Timer for ozone generator

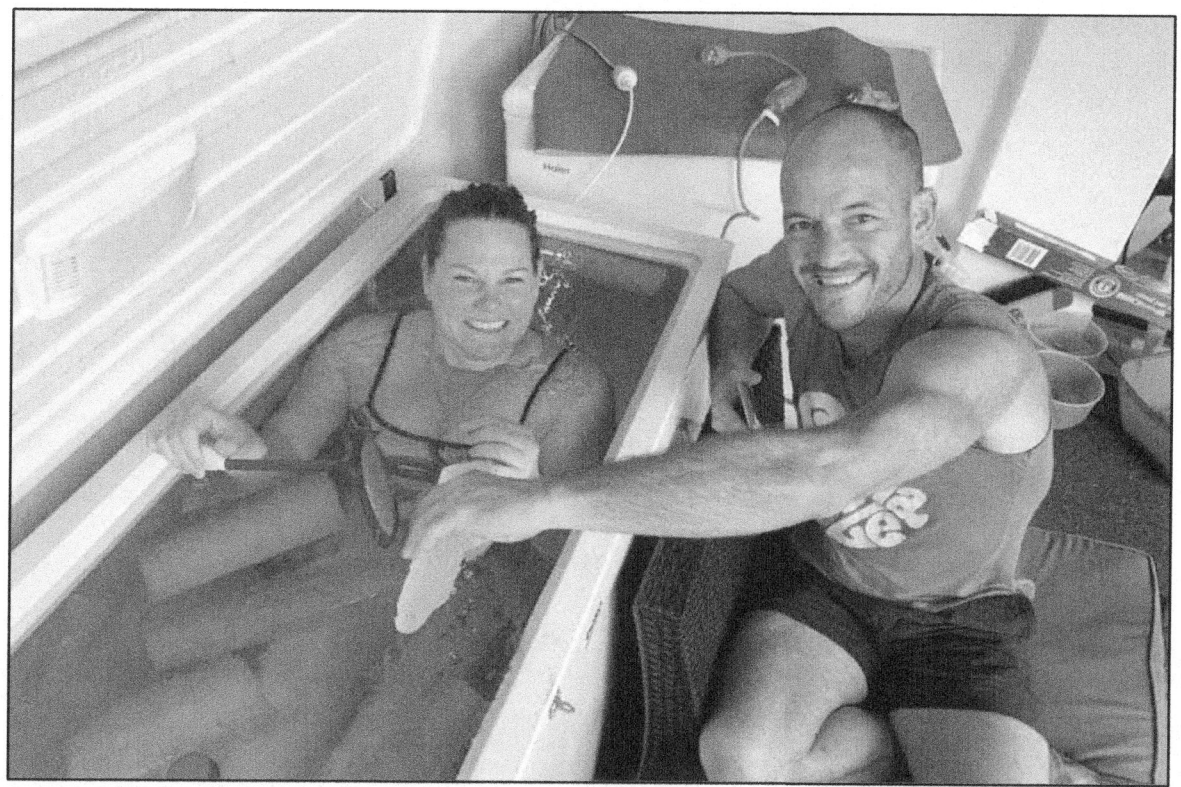

Tara Diversi & Michael Crawford, Australia

Brand: 500 L Beko

Location: Covered verandah

Seams: Sealed with Selly's wet area silicone

Water Sanitation: wash before getting in, 12kg salt, 30 mL spa clear

Initial chill: 4 days to go from 24° C to 8° C. Then threw in four 5 kg bags of ice.

Water Temp: Ranges from -1 to 2.5° C

Temperature Control: Outside power outlet with timer.

" " *Be daring, be different, be impractical;*
be anything that will assert integrity of purpose
and imaginative vision against the play-it-safers,
the creatures of the commonplace,
the slaves of the ordinary. " "

Cecil Beaton

Chapter 13:
Filling Your Chest Freezer

Now that you've sealed or lined your chest freezer, it is ready for water!

If possible, fill your chest freezer with softened or filtered water rather than tap water. If you don't have a water softener or filter, it is OK to use water from a standard garden hose. If there is a metal thread on the hose, be careful not to scratch or dent the inside of your chest freezer.

If you add too much water, you can use a small bucket to remove the excess.

PRE-FILTERS

The right filter on your garden hose can reduce sediment, odor, and chlorine. I use two filters. First is an inexpensive sediment filter, which extends the life of the second, more expensive filter.

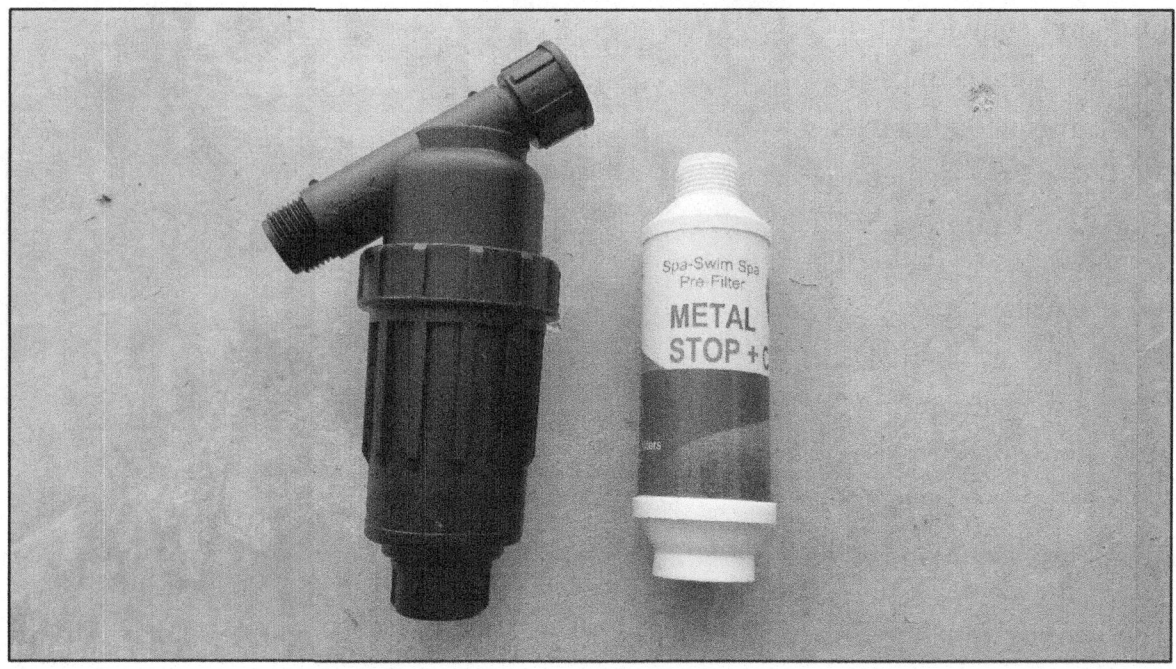

Mechanical filter (left), and spa filter (right)

Look for these filters in hardware stores near the parts for in-ground sprinkler systems. The mechanical filter should be the first filter that your water goes through.

The second filter is a chlorine filter. Chlorine eventually dissipates on its own. However, chlorine can dry out your skin, and some people are sensitive to the smell.

You may need a short hose to connect both filters.

TIP FOR APARTMENTS

If you live in an apartment or a place that does not have a hose bib, there are two options. The first is to buy an adapter for a garden hose that can attach to your kitchen sink. These adapters can range from $7 - $40.

The second option is a transfer pump and heavy-duty pump hose. Fill your bathtub about halfway with water and leave it running. Put the pump hose into the bathtub and connect it to the intake of the pump. Some pumps need to be primed. Read the owner's manual before starting.

If you use a standard garden hose for the intake, the pressure of the pump might collapse or break the hose. A standard garden hose for the discharge is OK.

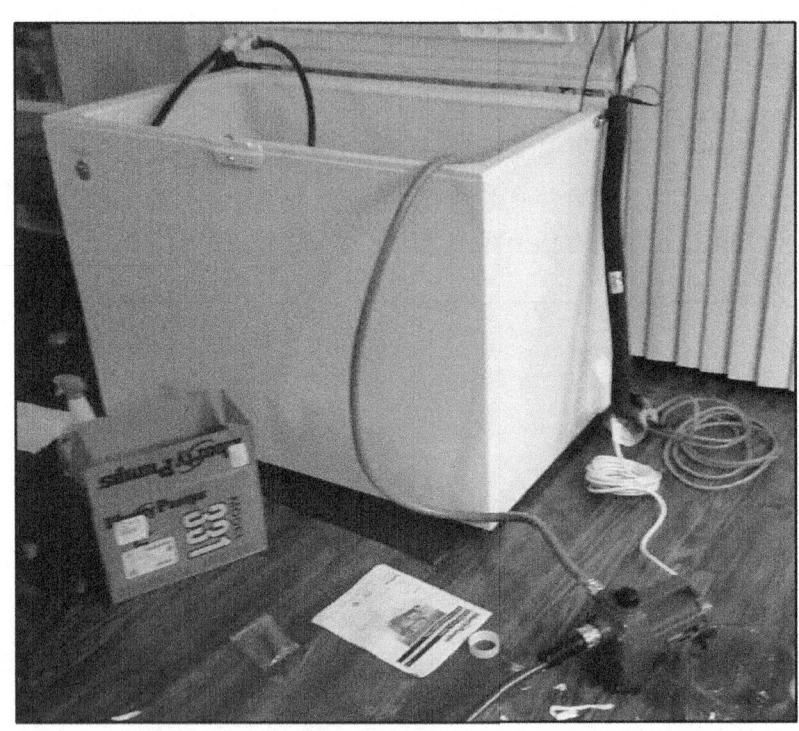

Transfer pump taking water from my bathtub to the freezer

It is best to use the long hose for the intake. Use a short hose to go from the pump to your cold tub.

HOW MUCH WATER TO ADD

Do not fill water to the top of your chest freezer. Plan for water displacement- just like in a bathtub.

Formulas for water displacement are complicated, so we will keep it simple. Start by leaving 6 - 8 inches (15 – 18 cm) from the top. When you get into your chest freezer, the water should be 1 - 2 inches (3 – 6 cm) below the plastic molding on the top wall.

If you sit on the floor of your chest freezer, it is best for the water to cover your shoulders. If it only goes up to your chest, you are missing out on some excellent physiological benefits. You have come this far – do not cheat yourself!

Now that you have everything set up and ready to go, your chest freezer is officially a cold plunge - congratulations!

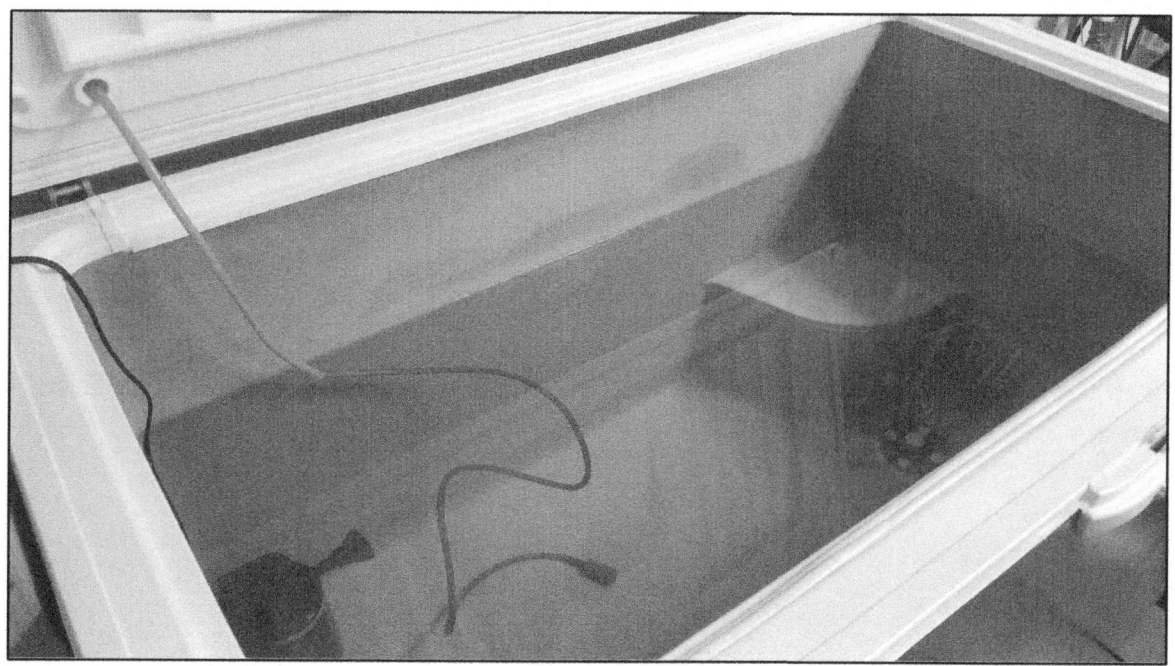

Water filled to 6-7 inches from the top wall

" *When we walk to the edge of all the light we have*
and take the step into the darkness of the unknown,
we must believe that one of two things will happen.
There will be something solid for us to stand
or we will be taught to fly. "

Patrick Overton

Chapter 14:
Chilling Your Water

It can take a few days for your chest freezer to chill the water to your target temperature. Depending on your ambient temperature, plan for 2 to 5 days.

While the chest freezer compressor is running, it is typical for the outside walls of the freezer to get very hot. They shouldn't get hot enough to burn you, but be careful. If you have children around, let them know to keep a safe distance.

 ## REDUCING YOUR COOLING TIME

If you want your water to chill faster, you can add crushed ice. See Appendix A to figure out how ice is needed. Add the ice first so you don't overfill your tub.

Adding enough salt to your water lowers the freezing point, which makes it cool faster. See the later section in this chapter on "Prevention."

 ## KEEPING YOUR WATER COLD

If you fill your chest freezer and leave it plugged in, you will end up with a solid block of ice. This not only makes cold water immersion impossible but is terrible for your chest freezer.

There are four ways to keep the water at your target temperature:

1. Plug / Unplug

This is the zero-budget option but requires the most amount of time and attention on your part. Each day, use a thermometer to measure the water temperature. If it starts to get too warm, plug in your chest freezer for a few hours. If it is too cold, unplug it for a few hours.

Many things can go wrong with this option, which is why I do not recommend it. If you forget or miscalculate the amount of time your freezer needs to be unplugged or plugged in, you won't have your ideal temperature.

2. Mechanical Timer

 A mechanical timer with a grounded plug makes it easier to keep the water at your target temperature. Timers can plug directly into an outlet but usually take up space, preventing another device from being plugged in. For that reason, use a short extension cord in between the timer and outlet. Refer to the connection diagram at the end of Chapter 7.

Plug your freezer into the controlled outlet on the timer. After you figure out how many hours your chest freezer needs to run each day, set the timer.

This setup saves you a lot of time and hassle. However, you still need to keep a close eye on it because there are a few potential problems:

As the ambient temperature changes, the time needed to cool your water changes.+

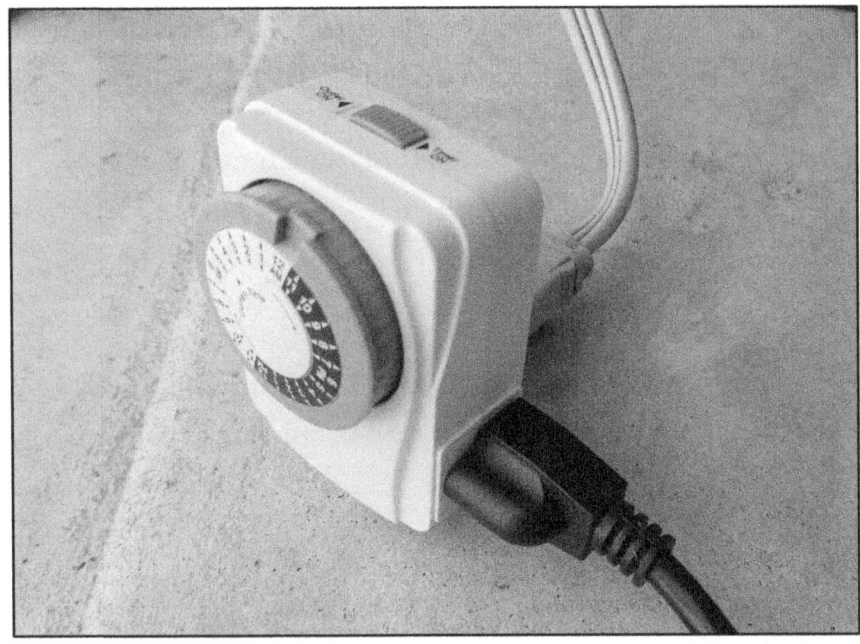

Mechanical Timer

When the power goes out (which it does each time you UNPLUG YOUR CHEST FREEZER before using it, right?), the run time of your timer changes. You can prevent this problem by getting a timer with a battery backup, or use smart home technology.

3. Smart Home Technology

If you already have a smart home set up, you can buy a smart plug and set it up to run on a schedule. This setup has the advantage of not needing to adjust the time manually. The main disadvantage is that if your setup depends on Wi-Fi and your internet is down, the timer won't work.

If you like this idea but do not want to spend the money setting up a smart home hub, X10.com sells digital home automation controllers and outlets that work through the wiring in your home.

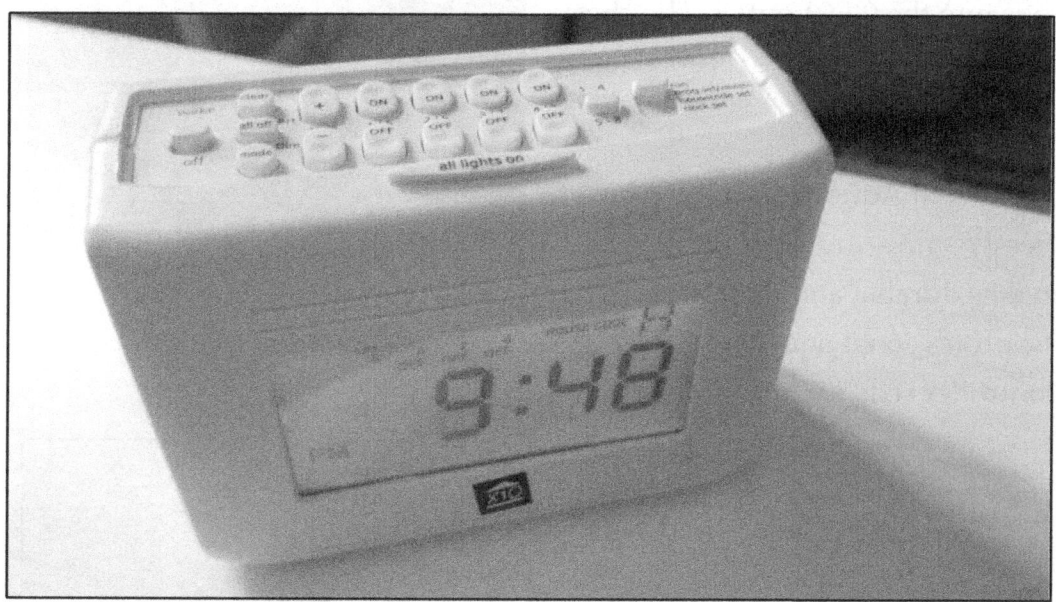

X-10 controller with clock

4. Temperature Controller

A temperature controller is the best way to maintain your water temperature. It has these advantages:

- The sensor turns the chest freezer power off and on according to the water temperature,

- You can set a high and low range

- Once you set it up, there is no need to fiddle with it

The sensor goes into the water, and the controller plugs into the GFCI outlet. The chest freezer power cord plugs into the receptacle outlet on the controller.

I use the Nema 4 from AquaLogic, which has worked flawlessly since August of 2017. AquaLogic makes durable and accurate equipment for professional aquariums. The AquaLogic controller sells for around $130.

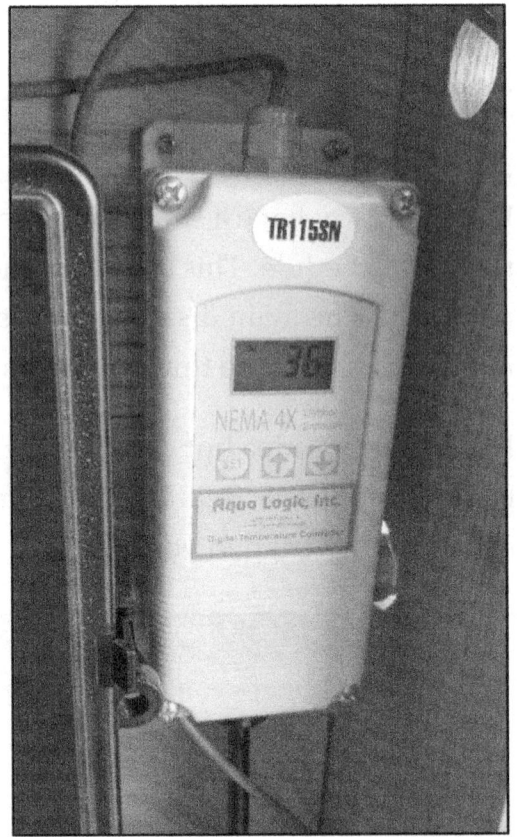

AquaLogic Nema 4 temperature controller

Many people have been happy with the less expensive InkBird controllers which sell for around $35.

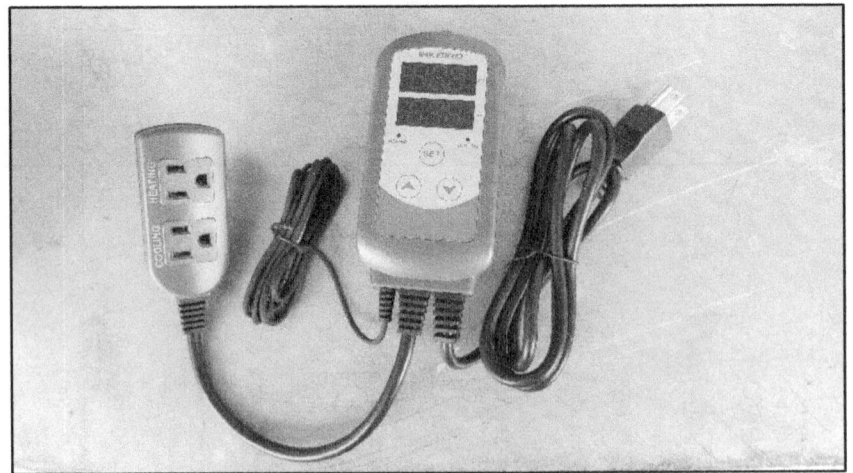

InkBird temperature controller

THE PROS AND CONS OF ICE BUILD-UP

Ice build-up in your cold plunge is expected. You will most likely see ice forming along the walls, on the water surface, and along the walls below the water surface.

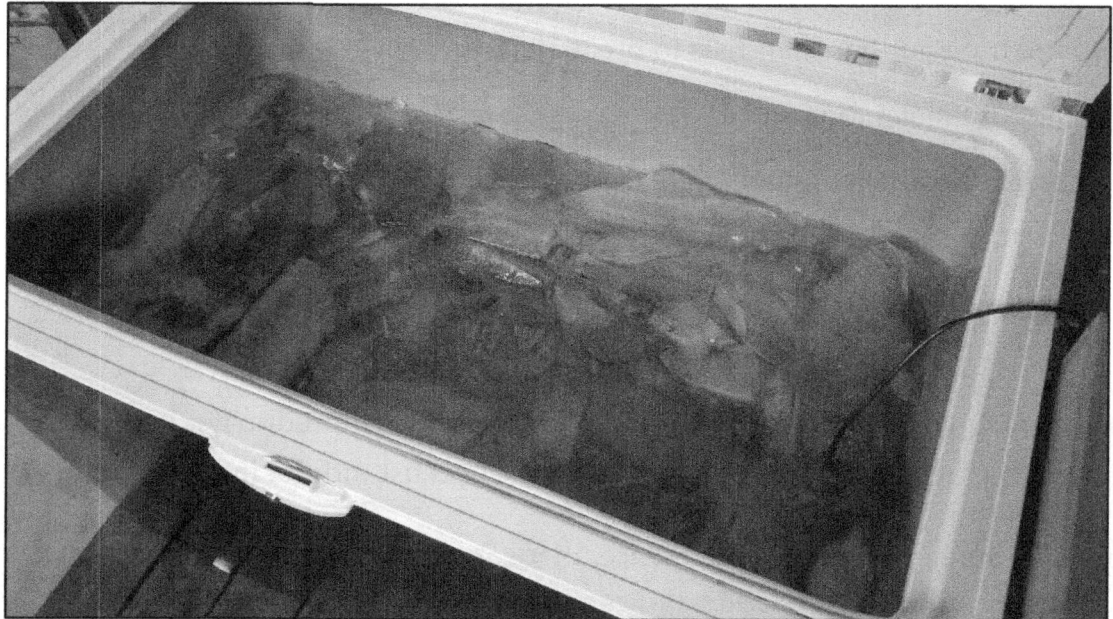

Too much ice!

There are some advantages to ice build-up. First, it keeps the water colder a little longer, which reduces the amount of time that your chest freezer compressor needs to run. Second, and most important, breaking through the ice water can bring a deep feeling of primal satisfaction.

However, there are some downsides.

1. Ice build-up makes your chest freezer compressor work harder than it needs to. Manufacturers recommend defrosting your chest freezer when 1/4" (.64 cm) of ice builds up on the walls.

2. Breaking the ice risks damaging your freezer or hurting yourself.

3. Larger pieces of ice, especially a ring around the edge, can make it dangerous for you to get in and out of the chest freezer. Broken ice can be sharp and could cut you.

4. If your skin is directly touching ice, there is an increased risk of frostbite.

BREAKING THE ICE

If you choose to let ice form in your chest freezer, there are a few safe ways to break it up.

1. Do not use your hands or fists to break the ice.

2. Do not use metal tools

3. To break the ice, use a tool made from rubber, plastic, or PVC, such as a mallet or 1" (2.5 cm) thick PVC pipe.

4. Avoid hitting the ice close to the wall

Prevention

After the novelty wore off, I grew tired of the extra work required to get into the cold plunge. Having one more thing on my to-do checklist did not improve my life.

If you would prefer not to deal with the ice, there are three solutions:

1. Install a submersible pump.

A submersible pump circulates the water, significantly reducing or preventing ice from building up.

Pond and fountain pumps/filters can also work.

Find a pump that has a flow rate of 2 – 3 times higher than the volume of water in your chest freezer. Any less is than that not enough. Too much more creates too much splashing.

We discussed pumps in more detail in Chapter 10.

2. Add salt to your water.

Adding salt to water lowers the freezing point, which reduces or eliminates ice buildup. The added benefit is that your compressor works less to chill the water, which extends the life of your chest freezer.

According to various chemistry and physics websites, a 10% salt solution lowers the freezing point of water to about 20° F (-6° C). Water at that temperature is much too cold for our purpose and is dangerous.

The Wim Hof Method recommends immersion in water between 32° – 40° F (0° – 4.4° C) for the most significant benefits.

How much salt is needed to lower the freezing point just enough for our purpose? That is a great question!

For our readers who are scientists or know the definition of "molality" and understand the formula for "freezing point depression" ($\Delta Tf = Kfm$)… you can figure this out on your own.

For the rest of us, a handy reference table is below for three standard chest freezer sizes. If you have a smaller or larger chest freezer, you can approximate how much salt to add or subtract.

Weight of Sodium Chloride (NaCl) Needed to Lower Freezing Point of Water

Target Freezing Point	Chest Freezer Size / Add This Much Salt		
	7-cu. ft. (198 L)	15-cu. ft. (424 L)	21cu. ft. (594 L)
30° F (-1.19° C)	6 lbs. / 2.9 kg	13 lbs. / 5.7 kg	18 lbs. / 8.2 kg
28° F (-1.79° C)	13 lbs. / 5.8 kg	25 lbs. / 11.4 kg	36 lbs. / 16.5 kg
26° F (-3.05° C)	16 lbs. / 7.2 kg	32 lbs. / 14.3 kg	45 lbs. / 20.6 kg

It takes more Epsom salts (MgSO4) than common salt (NaCl) to lower the freezing point. I could not find a formula for the exact amount, but you can add a little more.

Members from our group have reported using as little as 3 – 8 lbs. (1.4 – 3.6 kg) of Epsom salt to lower the freezing point enough to prevent ice buildup.
Note that salt may corrode metal in certain plastics. Refer to Appendix J: Chemical Compatibility.

3. Both of the above.
The third option is to use a pump and add salt.

Notes

_____

_____

_____

_____

_____

_____

_____

_____

_____

_____

_____

_____

_____

_____

_____

_____

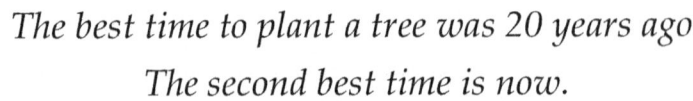

The best time to plant a tree was 20 years ago.
The second best time is now.

Chinese Proverb

Chapter 15:
Using Your Cold Plunge

In January 2016, I attended a workshop retreat for heart-centered entrepreneurs in Arizona. After dinner, several of us agreed to meet at the hot tub to connect and relax. The resort had a spacious cold plunge pool next to the hot tub. One of my friends said, "Let's see who can stay in the cold water the longest!"

I replied, "Let's see who can love themselves enough to get out when their body needs to!"

Cold water immersion is not a contest, and it's not really about how long you stay in the water. Wim Hof reminds us throughout his workshop, "No ego!"

As much as cold water immersion can benefit your body and mind, it can hurt you if you overdo it. Self-awareness is essential - know your limits! This chapter provides some insight into when to use and avoid using your chest freezer, as well as water temperatures and how long to stay in, however it is not a replacement for formal training.

I strongly recommend taking a live Wim Hof Method workshop. Also, check out this excellent e-book "A Practical Guide to Cold Training," by Jesse Coomer, who is a certified Wim Hof Instructor. Here is the link:

https://chestfreezercoldplunge.com/resources/

WHEN TO AVOID COLD WATER

It is recommended to *not* get into cold water if you:

- Have just eaten a large meal

- Completed a strength-training workout within the last 2-3 hours

- Are fasting

- Are sick

- Are under the influence of alcohol or drugs

- Feel exhausted or fatigued

- Have diarrhea

- Have an open wound (ex. from a cut, piercing, surgery) – unless covered with a waterproof bandage

- Have a medical condition or take medications that affect your body's ability to regulate temperature

- Have a critical illness, chronic disease or autoimmune issue unless you are under the guidance of a qualified health expert or a certified trainer (ex. Wim Hof Method) familiar with cold training protocols for health.

- Are in your ego, out to prove something, are showing off, or have not done enough research to be intelligent and safe in your approach.

◼ HYPOTHERMIA

Hypothermia happens when you get cold and your body cannot produce heat fast enough to warm yourself up. When your internal body temperature begins to drop below normal, hypothermia becomes dangerous. Cold water training, by its nature, creates some hypothermia. Too much can be dangerous.

There are several stages of hypothermia, each with particular symptoms. However, it is important to understand that because there can be extreme variations in responses to cold, these stages are listed for reference only.

1. **Mild:** shivering, increased blood pressure, fast heart rate or breathing, increased urine production

2. **Moderate:** confusion, slurred speech, loss of fine motor skills,

3. **Severe:** decreased heart rate, breathing rate, and blood pressure; lack of reflexes, hallucinations, fixed dilated pupils, confusion,

Because the symptoms begin gradually, they can be easy to miss. If you get to the second stage, reduced self-awareness can cause you to make bad decisions, such as not wanting to keep yourself warm and safe.

If you notice mild symptoms while in the water, it is time to get out. Build your tolerance slowly over time and do not push yourself. It is always better to err on the side of caution.

Staying in cold water too long can lead to frostbite, gangrene, and death.

It is always better to get out of cold water too soon than too late. However, one sign that you've stayed in too long is experiencing *afterdrop*.

AFTERDROP

When your core body temperature keeps dropping after you get out of cold water, this is known as *afterdrop*.

When you immerse yourself in cold water, your body keeps your organs warm by reducing blood flow to your skin, arms, and legs. When you get out of the cold water, cooler blood from your skin and limbs returns to your core and mixes with the warmer blood.

Symptoms of afterdrop are shivering or feeling colder than when you were in the water, feeling light headed, or unwell.

Afterdrop is not a sign of strength or progress, it is a symptom of a potentially serious or fatal condition and should be avoided. Err on the side of caution and train gradually and slowly.

If you experience afterdrop, it is best to warm yourself gradually. While you are still feeling cold, here are a few suggestions:

- Remove all wet clothes immediately.

- Dry off and put on warm clothes.

- Do horse stance, walk, or some other slow exercise.

- Sip a warm beverage and eat something.

- If you don't feel well, find a warm place to sit down.

- Do not take a hot shower or get in a sauna to warm yourself. Refer to the section later in this chapter on Contrast Therapy for exceptions to this rule).

- Do not drink alcohol or caffeine.

- Don't make important decisions

- Don't drive, ride a bike, or use a chainsaw.

CLEANLINESS IS NEXT TO...

Before you get into your chest freezer, it is a good idea to take a shower and wash your body with soap. Minimally, at least rinse off. The less sweat, skin flakes, and loose hair that you introduce into the water, the better.

Wear a swimsuit. I prefer speedo briefs over baggy shorts because more of your skin is exposed to cold water and there is way less dripping when you get out. Wearing a tight swimsuit also helps reduce/prevent fecal matter from getting into your water.

BREATHING AND HEATING YOURSELF UP

You can use the Wim Hof Method or another practice to prepare yourself to get into the cold water. It is ok to take a hot shower or sit in a sauna beforehand. Contrast therapy is discussed in more detail in the section at the end of this chapter.

TIME AND TEMPERATURE

There are different recommendations on how to get the most out of cold-water immersions.

When most people hear about cold water immersion, they think of ice baths used by athletes. Coaches and spas use ice baths, or cold plunges typically set at around 57° F (13.9° C).

Certified Wim Hof Method (WHM) trainers agree that for most people, 2 - 3 minutes in water between 32 - 40° F (0° - 4.4° C) to () provides optimal benefits. Staying in water for more than three minutes seems to have diminishing returns for most people.

There are exceptions to this, and if you have questions, take a Wim Hof Method course or get coaching from a certified trainer.

I set the water in my chest freezer to range between 34 – 36° F (1.1 – 2.2 C). I like this range because it gives me a margin of error.

Some people set their water temperature lower; however, temperatures at or less than 32° F (0° C) can cause frostbite and increase your risk of hypothermia.

Water temperature below freezing is not recommended!

Large population quantified data (scientific research) on the human physiological response to various temperatures of cold water does not yet exist. I have a vision of someday setting up a cold-water research laboratory to collect this data.

As far as we know now, there does not seem to be a significant benefit to plunging into water colder than freezing- 32° F (0° C). Temperatures below freezer bring significant risks and are not recommended.

What about temperatures above 40° F (4.4° C)? You can definitely benefit, but it seems to take longer immersion times. Some people like to start at warmer temperatures, building their tolerance slowly, and gradually working down to colder temperatures.

Some people enjoy spending 20 - 45 minutes in water that is 50° F (10° C). Others prefer water at 32° F (0° C). It's up to you! A chest freezer makes all of this not only possible but manageable.

There has been recent discussion about the benefits of changing your scheduling to alternate temperatures from near-freezing up to is 50° F (10° C).

Essential parts of a cold training program include preparing yourself to get into the water, what to do while in the water, and what to do afterward. It is beyond the scope of this guide to provide details about safe and effective cold training programs; however, here are a few guidelines.

Real World Setup

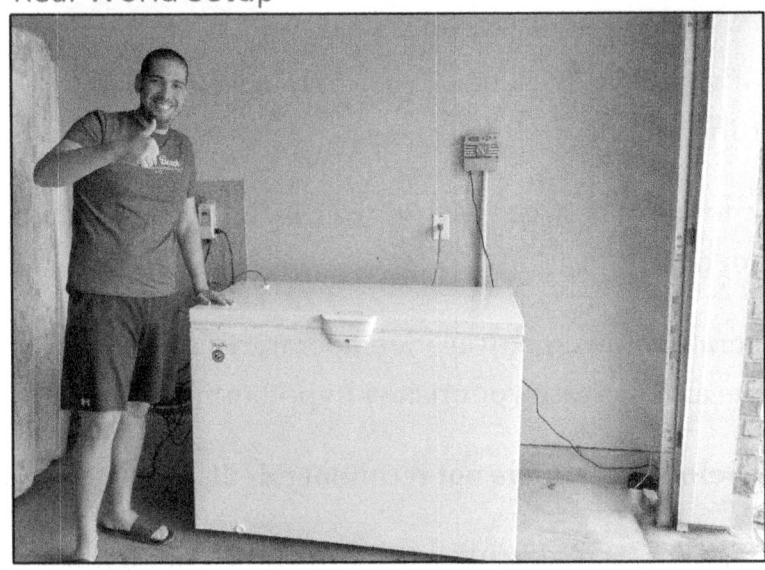

Paulo R.'s cold plunge in Austin, TX

Brand / Size: Whirlpool 15-cu. ft. (424 L)

Location: Garage

Seams: Sealed with JB Water Weld

Water Sanitation: MarineLand aquarium pump/filter, JED Ozone Generator (2 hours per day), change the water once every 60 days

Temp: 39° F (3. 9° C)

Temperature Control: AquaLogic

Training Protocol: 2 – 3 times per week

If I had to do it again: Would buy a larger chest freezer

◼ TRAINING PLAN

Peter Turla, a former NASA rocket designer, said: "It is better to do the right thing slowly than the wrong thing quickly." This philosophy applies to cold water training.

In the absence of having a trained coach or teacher, gradual acclimation to cold water is the best approach. Besides your breathing and mindset, there are two things that you can control:

1. The water temperature, and

2. How long you stay in the water.

Each person responds and adapts to cold on their schedule. Pay attention to your body, and build gradually. If your goal is to be in cold water for 2 minutes and your body starts shivering after 30 seconds, get out!

Some people recommend starting with cold showers. Alternate between hot and cold, but always end on cold. Increase the time you spend in the cold water.

With the cold plunge, start with warmer temperatures and shorter times. A 1-degree change in water temperature can cause a significant mental and physical response. Go slow!

Here are some ideas to get you started.

◼ Frequency of Training

How often should you get into cold water?

- It is OK to train each day as long as your body responds well. Others train one to three times a week or just once a week.
- You can train more than once per day. Do not get back into cold water on the same day until your body has warmed up.
- It is OK to take time off as needed. Pay attention to your body.
- The best results come with consistency over time (months or years).
- It still useful to take daily cold showers.

▣ Progressions

There is a Training Log in Appendix M. Record your sessions each day so you can see your progress. Make notes about how you feel and how your body responds while in the water and afterward. Set a goal. If you don't know what goal to set, work toward 2 - 3 minutes in water at or below 40° F (4.4° C).

You can create your own training plan, but here is an example.

For each temperature, start with 30 seconds. Build time gradually. Go for 1 minute, then 2, and 3.

At temperatures above 50° F (10° C) you can work up to 10 minutes or longer times if your body is responding well. This means no shivering, burning or tingling while in the water, and no shivering or after drop after getting out.

After you are comfortable at 10 minutes, lower your temperature and start over with 30 seconds. You can lower your temperature 4 to 6 1 degrees at a time, or 2 degrees at a time. Slow is better.

If you have a hard time at a lower temperature, it's perfectly OK to go back to warmer water.

At temperatures below 40°F (4.4° C), the WHM recommends staying in for no more than 2-3 minutes. However, people have reported being OK staying in longer.

Keep in mind that there are no real data or evidence-driven levels, and these temperatures are for reference.

Level 1	Level 2	Level 3
65°F (18.3° C)	50°F (10° C)	36°F (2.2° C)
60°F (15.5° C)	45°F (7.2° C)	34°F (1.1° C)
55°F (12.8° C)	40°F (4.4° C)	32°F (0° C)

MORNING, NOON, OR NIGHT?

Most people recommend doing cold training first thing in the morning before you eat. It is okay to drink some water first.

If early morning does not work for your schedule, the next best time is during the day.

Third best is at night. However, keep in mind that getting into cold water within 2 - 3 hours of bedtime might disrupt your sleep.

If you have insomnia, cold water immersion before bed might give you a *great* night's sleep, but you have to play around with the timing, temperature, and duration to dial it in.

 ## PREPARATION FOR COLD WATER IMMERSION

There are two schools of thought about what to do before you get in, and both have their merits.

The first school of thought is to prepare yourself with breathing, stretching, or some form of exercise or formal practice to generate heat in your body. These techniques can be learned in the Wim Hof Method.

The second school of thought is to not prepare yourself, and notice how your body responds naturally.

 ## GETTING INTO YOUR COLD PLUNGE

Place a microfiber bath mat on the floor in front of your chest freezer. Wear house shoes or flip flops to the freezer to keep your feet clean and wipe them on the mat before getting in. The less dirt you track into the chest freezer, the easier it is to keep clean.

A small step in front makes it easier to climb into and out of the chest freezer. If you are tall, this may not be an issue.

Keep the chest freezer locked when not in use. I have a small magnet on the side that I use to hold the key. Unlock your chest freezer and open the lid first. Glance at the water and make sure it looks clean and that the filter is running. Then unplug everything from the power source.

Place a small towel or washcloth over the locking mechanism to prevent water from splashing inside and causing rust.

Get in purposefully and with deliberation. Do not go so fast that you splash or cause waves, but do not get in too slowly. Aim to immerse yourself with water over your shoulders in less than 10 seconds from the time you step in.

I like to inhale as I step in, and exhale as I set down. Exhaling helps avoid the gasp reflex. Experiment to discover what works best for you.

Real World Setup

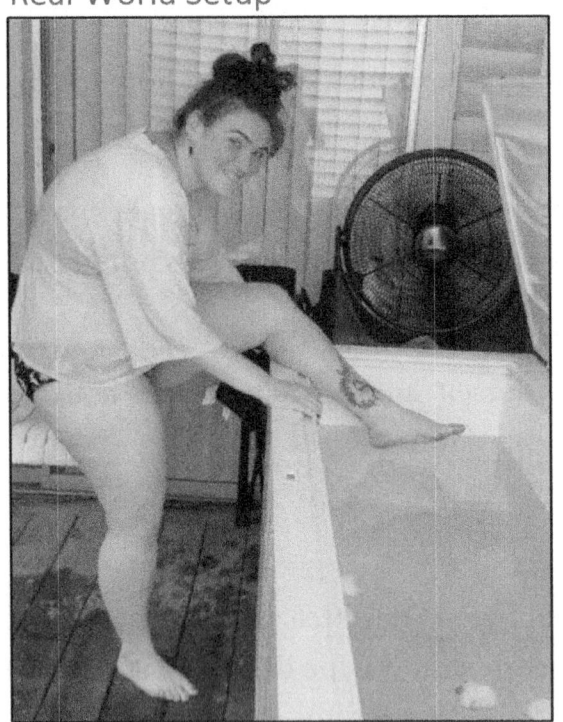

Photo courtesy of John Patterson, Houston, TX

Chest Freezer: 21-cu. ft. Frigidaire, used

Water Temp: 32° F (0° C)

Location: Covered patio

Sealed with: JB Water Weld (all underwater seams), silicone (above water)

Water Sanitation: Pond filter and UV sterilizer. 1 tbsp. laundry bleach per week + partial water change (30%) as needed

What didn't work: Applied 5 coats of Flex Seal to scratches on the inside, and they rusted in a few weeks

■ Cold Shock

"Cold Shock" is the physiological response to sudden immersion in cold water. Symptoms include a gasping of breath and an intense feeling of panic. Some medical literature states that this response is involuntary and automatic. Most reports of death due to cold water exposure, indicate drowning as the cause- not hypothermia- because the initial cold shock causes people to inhale water.

However, from direct experience, we know this is not the case. It is possible to overcome the cold shock response through proper preparation before getting into cold water or through conditioning.

 ## WHILE IN THE TUB: YOUR COLD PRACTICE

Sit on the floor of the cold plunge. Do not sit on the thing that looks like a seat (the compressor cover) because it was not built to handle the weight. Many people find that having the water come up over their shoulders gives an overall better experience.

Sit with your knees bent, and feet flat on the floor in front of you. You can put your back against the side wall. I like to rest the top back of my head on the top edge of the wall, which keeps my back away from the wall and exposed to the cold. On top of that, it gets my neck and the lower back of my head underwater, which some say is good for the vagus nerve.

■ Mindfulness

Relax all of your muscles. The more you relax, the better your body will respond to the cold. If you find yourself tensing up certain muscles, it's OK. Just relax. The more you practice, the easier it becomes.

I usually prefer to keep still while in the water. However, some people like to move slowly to keep the thin layer of water over their skin from heating up. It's up to you. Just be sure to use slow movements that don't cause waves or splashing.

While in the cold water, do NOT practice the Wim Hof breathing (specifically breath retention) because there is a risk of passing out.

You may find that slow, deep breaths are helpful. I find that inhaling for 5 seconds and exhaling for 5 seconds is helpful. Sometimes my breathing is even slower. Being in cold water is an excellent place to practice mindfulness.

■ Hands and Feet

Some people keep their hands out of the water; others put them in right away or put them in for only part of the session. If you find your hands getting too cold, take them out of the water.

You may benefit from doing hand isolation exercises, which is placing just your hands up to the wrists or elbows into the water. You can learn more about this practice in the Wim Hof Method courses or on the Wim Hof Method Facebook group.

Some people do separate training for their feet. For that purpose, it is OK to step in and just stand in the chest freezer. Do not sit on the side walls because it isn't safe and puts strain on the seams.

■ Is Your Chest Freezer Still Plugged In?

If you remember or notice that your chest freezer is still plugged in, take the advice of the late Douglas Adams and "Don't Panic!" Get out slowly and deliberately, using the steps mentioned in the "When and How to Get Out" section later in this chapter.

The good news is that some people have reported being in their chest freezer cold plunge while it was still plugged in – me included – and we have lived to tell about it. This is not a valid rationale to leave it plugged in, but mentioned only to give reassurance you if you forget.

At the PachaMama Eco-Community in Costa, Rica, Yati Or invites newcomers to their first cold water immersion. He keeps the temperature of his cold plunge at 46° F (8°C) and encourages people to stay in for at least one minute.

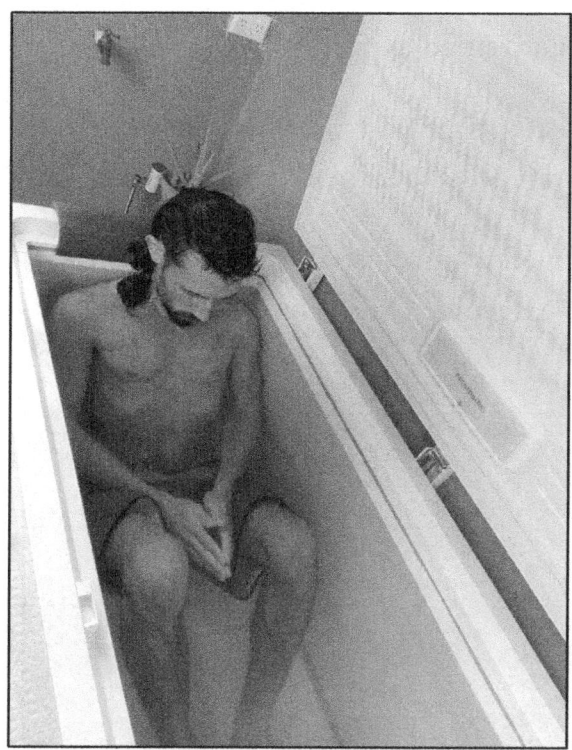

Yati Or, Costa Rica

■ Mindfulness Check List

Mindfulness is bringing your attention/focus to what is happening in the present moment. Accept whatever is happening without judging it.

There are a few things to notice that can help you be mindful while in cold water

1. Notice your breathing

2. Be aware of how the water feels against your skin

3. Notice your thoughts and emotions

4. Find and release any tension in your body

■ Head Dunking

There are differing opinions on the benefits of dunking your head. That conversation is beyond the scope of this guide. However, if you do wish to dunk your head, here are a few suggestions:

1. Do your research and get coaching from a trained expert!

2. It is best to dunk your head while the rest of your body is in the water. Dunking your head only in cold water may lead to loss of consciousness.

3. Cold water can be tough on your eyes, even when closed. Some people find it helpful to wear goggles and swimmer's earplugs. Others like to add nose plugs and swim caps.

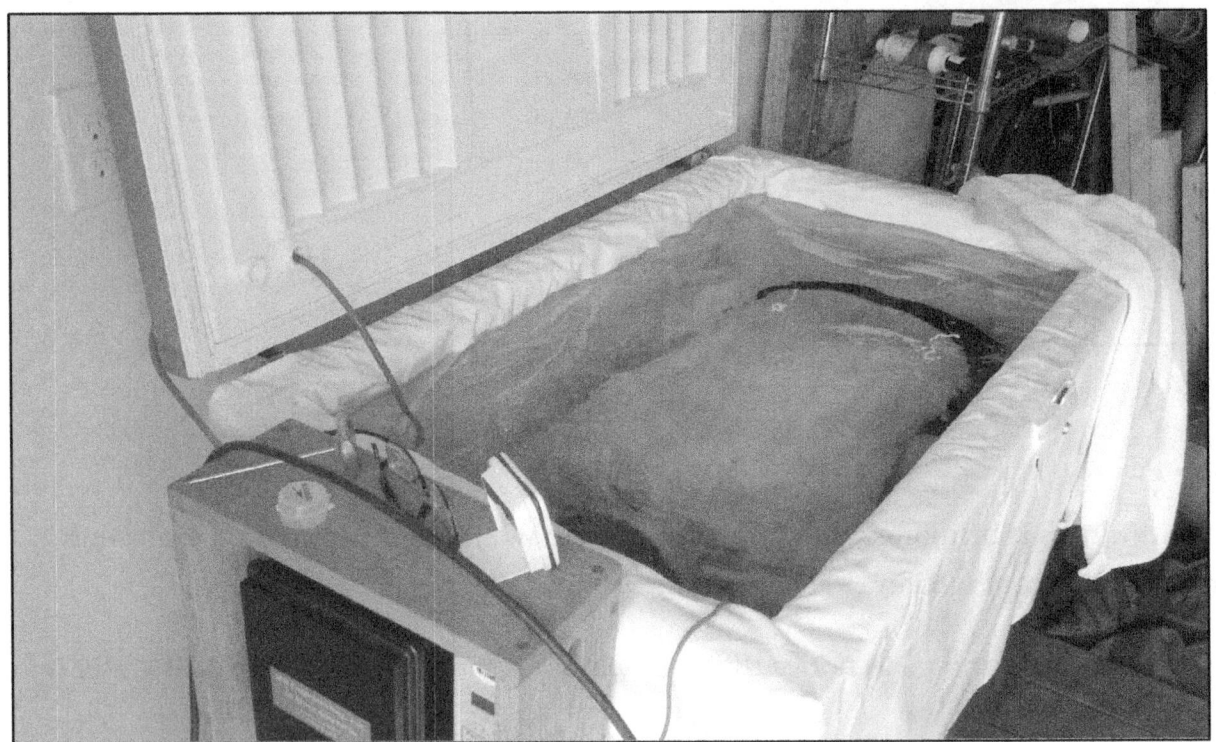

Head dunk from a kneeling position

4. I found that starting in a kneeling position and submerging my entire body is most comfortable. I press against one side wall with my feet and the opposite wall with my hands to hold myself underwater. Others scooch their butt forward and lean back, dunking their head from the sitting position.

5. Holding your breath on the inhale is recommended. Do not hold your breath on the exhale because there is risk of blacking out. Hyperventilating is not recommended while in the water.

6. Do not use snorkels or any other kind of breathing apparatus to keep yourself underwater longer than you can naturally hold your breath.

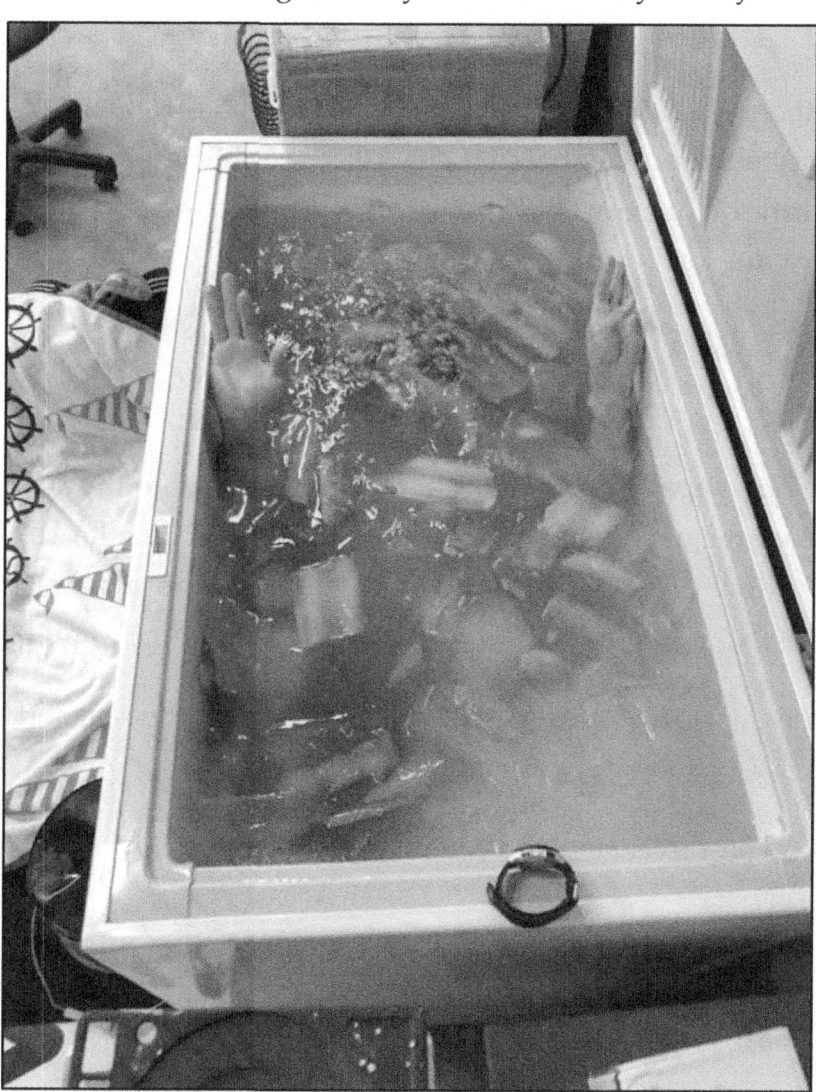

Derek D. head dunking from a sitting position

WHEN AND HOW TO GET OUT

Wim Hof trainers say that for most people, two to three minutes in cold water gives you the most significant benefit. If you stay in longer than that, there is a diminishing return. In other words, staying in longer than 3 minutes does not give you enough additional benefit to be worth the time spent. Set a countdown timer, but use it as a reference only, not as a goal.

As Wim Hof reminds us, this is not about ego, but about trusting your body.

Always pay attention to your body. If you feel numbness, burning, tingling, or start to shiver – get out!

Stand up slowly and deliberately. Try not to splash water. I keep a towel within reach and like to dry off as much as I can before I get out of the chest freezer. This gives my feet and legs a little bit of extra cold-training. If your feet and legs are not comfortable with the extra time, get out!

AFTER YOU GET OUT

Taking Care of Your Cold Plunge
After you are completely out, wipe off any water that has splashed onto the lid and tops of the walls. Also check the outside walls, especially the back above the compressor. If water leaks down the back wall and gets onto the compressor or into that area, it can start to rust.

Lock the chest freezer when you are done using it. Locking tightens the seal and makes it kid-safe.

Remember to plug in your chest freezer!

Taking Care Your Body

Pay close attention to your body. Expect your skin to be red or flushed. Bluish skin is not ok and indicates that you stayed in too long.

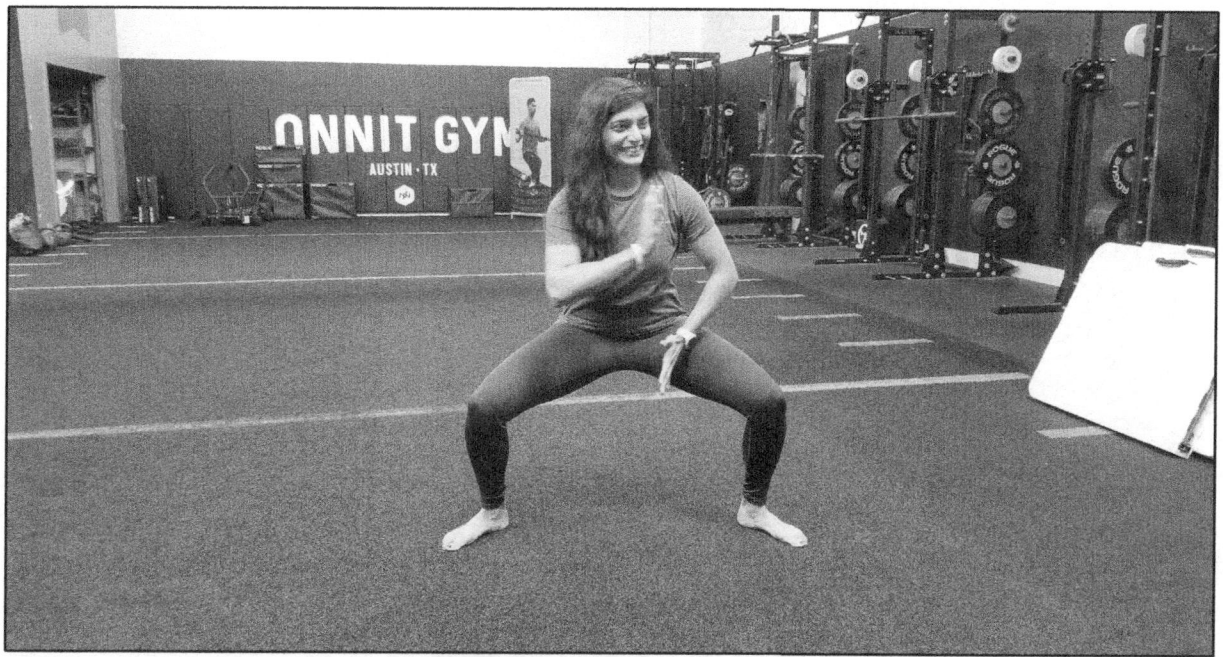

Shereen Yusuff, a certified WHM instructor, demonstrating horse stance

If you have a post-cold exposure practice, you can do that now.

Spend a few minutes in horse stance, controlling your breathing. Hose stance is a great way to warm your body and can help prevent afterdrop. Walking, qi-gong, and tai chi can also be helpful.

Vigorous exercise is not recommended. Wait until your body warms up before you go jogging, lift weights, or do calisthenics.

The main thing we want to look out for is something known as *afterdrop*, which was discussed earlier in this chapter.

■ Memory Tips for Plugging and Unplugging

It is easy not to remember to unplug or plug in your power cord, and most of us have done this at one time or another. However, it is also straightforward to set up a system to help you remember.

1. Ritual

As part of your "Entry Ritual" always unplug your chest freezer. After you finish, always plug in your chest freezer. Make it a habit. Consciously think about it as part of your mindfulness practice.

2. Everywhere a Sign

Some people post a sign on the wall above their chest freezer to help jog their memory. Paulo R. made this sign:

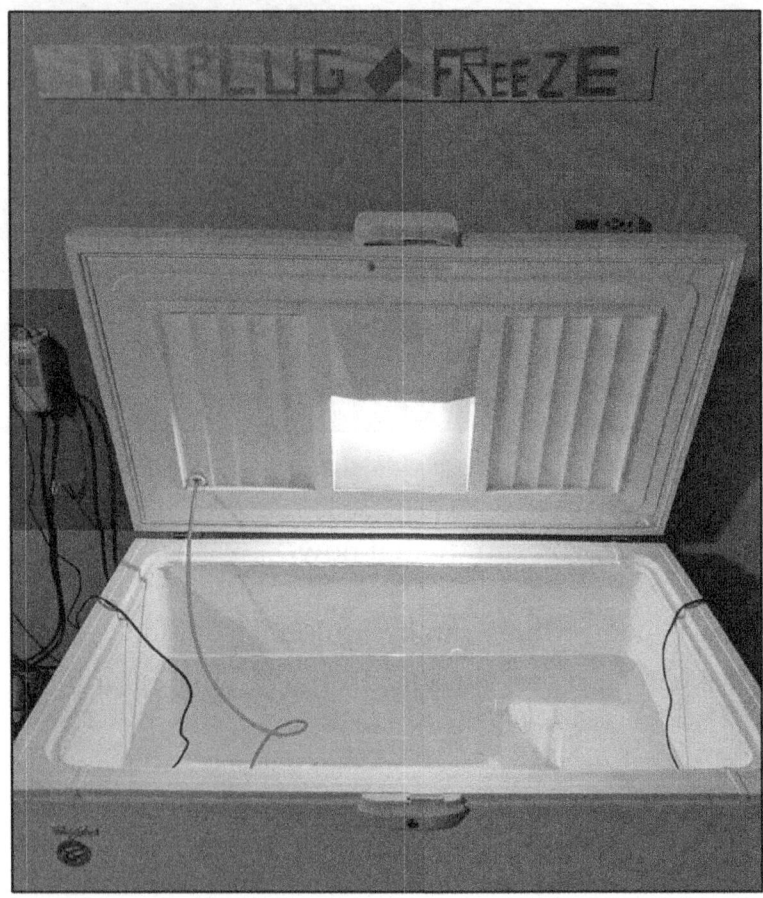

Reminder sign

3. Look at the Light

This tip is helpful unless you are using a temperature controller or timer, which might turn off power to your chest freezer when it is still plugged in. If you are not using a timer or temperature controller, look at the light before you get in. If it is on, unplug the chest freezer! After you finish, make sure the light is back on before you close the lid.

4. Power Cord as a Lock

Lars F., who lives in Sweden, rigged it so that his lid cannot open without unplugging the power. The power cord is attached to the lid with a few screws and is attached to an extension cord. Be careful not to get the outlet wet.

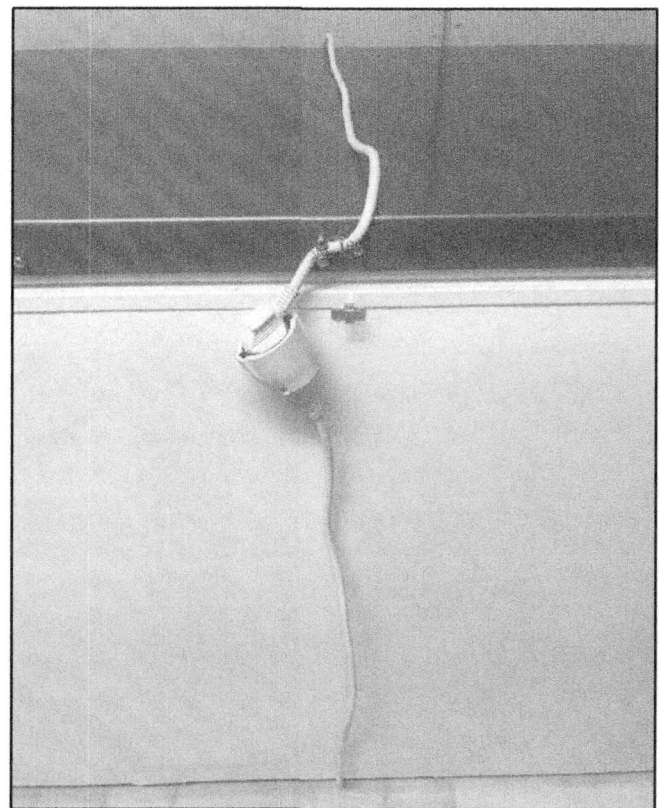

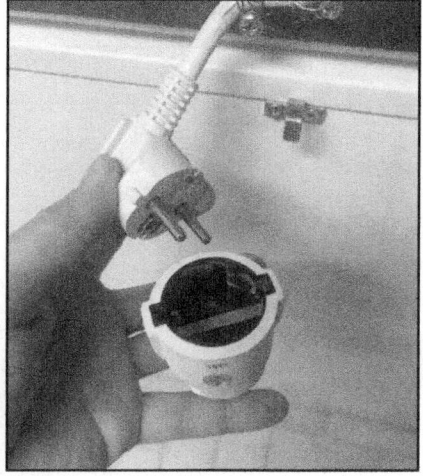

Unplugged = unlocked

The power cord lock plugged in

5. Smart Home Option

Alan R. installed a Smart Home contact sensor on side of the lid and side wall of his chest freezer. It is similar to the switches used in home security systems for doors and windows. Whenever the lid opens, the sensor breaks contact and turns off the power automatically. A smart home sensor can be a useful backup in case you forget to turn off the power.

However, to remove 100% of the risk, the power cord must be completely unplugged from the outlet.

◼ CONTRAST THERAPY

In 2014 I visited Orr Hot Springs in northern California. We spent the day lounging between the hot springs at 108° F (42.2° C) and the 60°F (15.6° C) spring-fed pool.

I found that to be one of the most relaxing days I've ever experienced.

Contrast therapy is going back and forth between hot and cold temperatures. If you have access to a hot tub, sauna, steam room, or even a bathtub filled with hot water, you can alternate between heat and cold water.

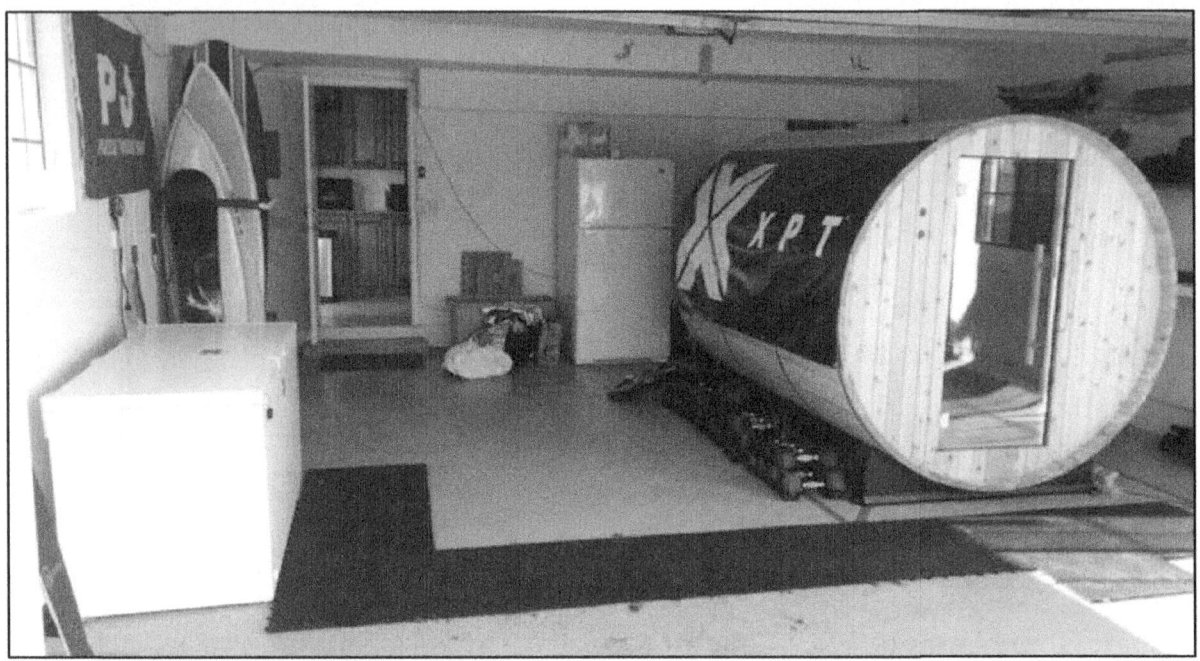

Mike Rut's chest freezer and sauna setup in Newport Beach, CA

Contrast therapy is reputed to have excellent health benefits, including:

- Reduced pain
- Improved circulation
- Reduced muscle soreness
- Increased energy
- Improved mood

There are few scientific studies, but recent research indicates that contrast therapy may improve levels of glutathione, which is an antioxidant produced by your body.

◼ Suggested Protocols

There are many ways to enjoy contrast therapy. Here are a few tips:

- Start with heat.

- Alternate between the two for 15 – 30 minutes.

- You can stay in the heat and cold for equal amounts of time or stay in the heat longer. Typical ratios of heat to cold (in minutes) are 1:1 up to 5:1.

- Do not apply heat to recent injuries that are swollen or red.

- Always end with cold water.

As with cold training, there are potential risks to contrast therapy. Pay attention to your body and do not push for time. Be sure to drink enough water.

"*The way must be in you;*
the destination also must be in you
and not somewhere else in space or time.

If that kind of self-transformation
is being realized in you, you will arrive."

Thic Nhat Hanh

Chapter 16: Maintenance

Performing regular maintenance keeps your chest freezer up and running more often, extends its life, and gives you more time to enjoy your cold-water immersion with fewer interruptions.

There is a maintenance log in Appendix L. Here are a few things you can record:

- The date you set up your chest freezer

- Equipment used

- Starting water temperature

- Target water temperature

- # of days to chill

- The date you add new equipment

- The date and details when you change your process or setup (ex. added 8 lbs./3.6 kg of Epsom salts; or installed ozone generator)

- Problems/issues

Keeping meticulous notes helps you troubleshoot problems.

Always unplug everything before doing any cleaning or maintenance!

How much and what kind of maintenance you need to do depends on several variables, but mostly on the environment where you have your chest freezer and how you sanitize your water.

 ## GENERAL CLEANING

Once a week, wipe the inside walls with a soft kitchen sponge. You don't need to use soap.

Use a fine mesh fish net to scoop out hair or other stuff floating in the water.

If you have a filter, clean it on a regular schedule. Start by checking it once a week. If it is clean, add another week. You might find that cleaning the filter once every 3 – 4 weeks is sufficient. Don't go for more than one month.

Keep a second filter handy and alternate it each month. It is easier to remove hair and dirt when the filter is dry. After cleaning, store it in a closed box to keep it from getting dusty.

Some people use a mini hot tub vacuum. I bought one that works like a giant straw but rarely use it because I'm diligent about wiping my feet before I get in.

Wipe the outside walls at least every week or two.

Once per month, check the compressor compartment for dust or cobwebs. UNPLUG the cold plunge before cleaning the mechanics. These parts can get hot, and there is a risk of shock or electrocution. Be careful not to bend or break anything.

It is better to use compressed air or a vacuum to clean the mechanics rather than wiping them or using a broom.

 ## TESTING YOUR WATER

Keeping your water clean is essential. The only way to know with 100% certainty that your water is clean is to test it. However, most people I've talked with do not formally test their water. If you see cloudy water or smell an odor, it is past time to change it.

The danger of relying on observation alone is that microorganisms may be in your water even if it is crystal clear and odor-free.

One downside to traditional testing is that the solutions to fix the problems identified (ex. with pH or total alkalinity) require standard pool chemicals.

Chlorine, bromine, and other typical pool and spa products can cause skin irritation, have strong odors and contain ingredients that some people consider to be toxic. These concerns inspire people to consider alternative sanitation products and methods such as ozone and hydrogen peroxide.

It is beyond the scope of this guide to go into detail about standard spa chemicals; however, if you want to go this route, there is an overview.

For specific product recommendations, consult your local spa and swimming pool supply store. The levels mentioned below are ranges and averages from the various pool and spa experts. You'll need to find the ideal range for your water.

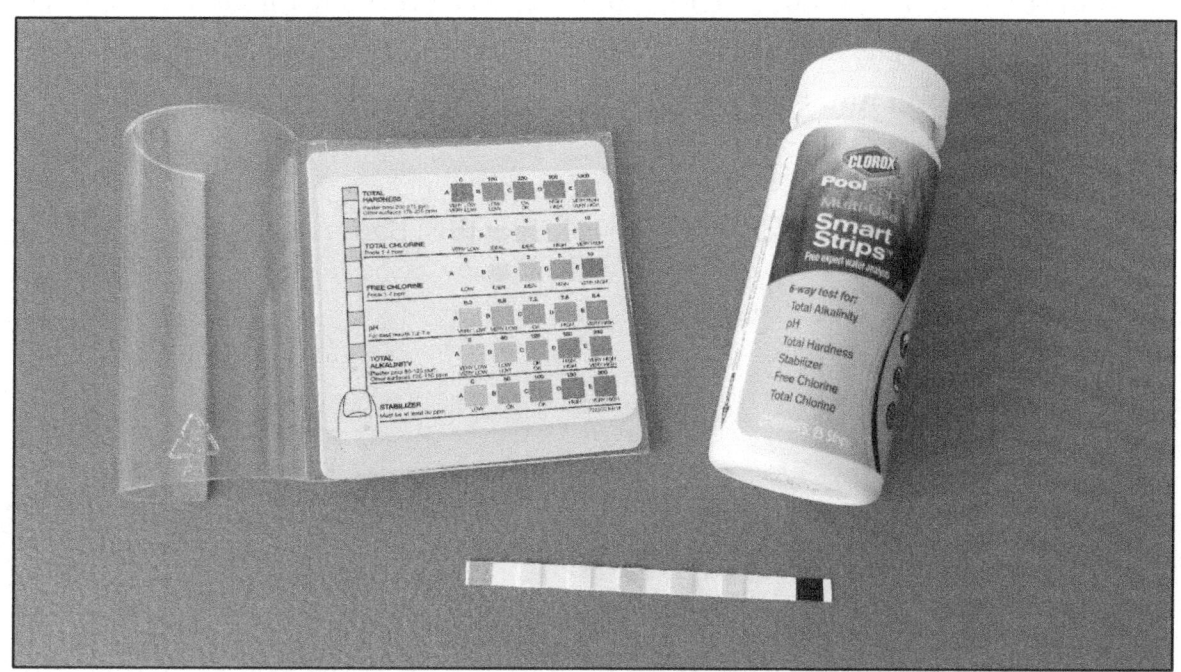

Pool and spa test strips

Water testing kits can be purchased online or from local spa & pool suppliers.

Some test kits work with an app that you download to your phone; however, this is unnecessary.

Some pool supply stores provide a small container that you can fill with water to bring back for free testing. You can buy strips and digital kits that test many aspects of your water. Here are a few key things to test:

1. Total Alkalinity

Total alkalinity (TA) is considered to be the most crucial test for hot tub owners. TA affects and helps you control the pH of your water, so it must be adjusted before you test or adjust your pH. If the TA is off, you won't get correct results with your pH test.

TA should range between 80 – 150 PPM.

Chemicals can be added to bring the TA up or down as needed.

Always test and balance TA before you move on to pH.

2. pH

pH is the measure of how acidic or basic your water is. The scale ranges from 0 to 14. As you go down the scale, each lower number is 10 times more acidic than the number above it. Lower numbers are more acidic. Higher numbers are more basic. 7 is neutral.

If that doesn't make sense, think of the pH scale like this: Battery acid

0	Gastric acid
1	Vinegar
2	Orange juice
3	Tomato juice
4	Black coffee
5	Urine
6	Distilled water
7	Eggs
8	Baking soda
9	Milk of magnesia
10	Ammonia
11	Soapy water
12	Bleach
13	Liquid drain cleaner

Items at the top and bottom of the scale are caustic.

When your pH is either too high or too low, here are potential problems: unsanitary water (bacteria)

- staining

- skin and eye irritation

- cloudy water

- corrosion

- deterioration of plastic components

Water pH should measure between 7.2 and 7.8.

If pH is either too high or too low, different products are required to increase or decrease it.

3. Calcium Hardness

Calcium hardness, also known as "total hardness," measures the level of calcium and magnesium in water. Here are some symptoms that can show up when your hardness is too low or high:

- foam

- scale

- corrosion

- deterioration of the metal components

- cloudy water

Ideal calcium readings differ depending on the spa's material. Since your cold plunge isn't made from standard spa or pool materials (acrylic or plaster), I can only guess what the reading should be. 100 – 450 is the standard range for spas.

If your calcium level is too high, products can be added to prevent scale; however, no chemical can lower the calcium levels. The ideal solution is to fill your cold plunge with water that has been through a softener if one is available. If not, it will be ok.

If you have low calcium readings, you can add a calcium booster.

4. Bacteria

The biggest concern about water sanitation is bacteria and microorganisms. It is possible for your water to be crystal clear with no odor and still have bacteria in it. This is one additional reason to avoid head-dunking in your cold plunge unless you are the only one using it and have impeccable hygiene.

Standard pool test kits do not test for bacteria. Most simple DIY bacteria test kits only test for E. coli and coliform. The only way to test your water for all bacteria is to send it to a lab, which is expensive and can take a few weeks.

It is up to you as to whether or not you choose to test for bacteria.

Real World Setup

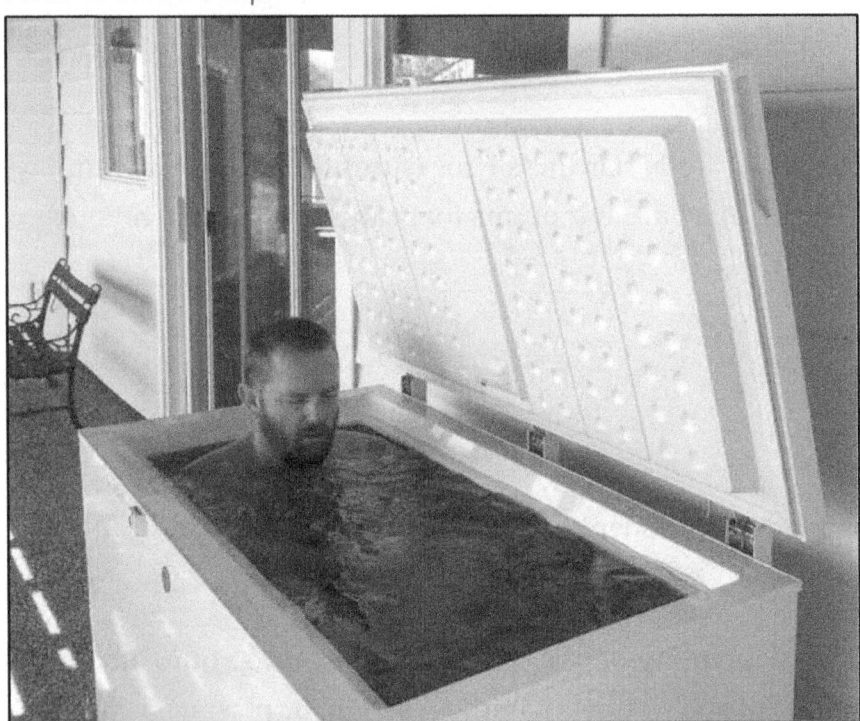

Justin I.'s setup in Arizona, USA

Size: GE 10.6-cu. ft. (300 L)

Location: Garage

Seams: Sealed with JB Water Weld

Water Sanitation: Aquamarine pump

TEST YOUR GFCI

GFCI outlets typically work reliably for many years. However, it is possible for them to fail and lose their safety function.

Once per month, test your GFCI to make sure that it is working. Push the Test button with your finger. You should hear a snapping sound that trips the outlet and cut off the power. An easy way to determine if the power is off is to plug a lamp or radio into the outlets and make sure they do not turn on. After you perform the test, press the reset button.

If the GFCI fails, do not plug anything back in and replace it as soon as possible.

WHEN TO CHANGE YOUR WATER

When do you need to change your water? There are a few signs. If your water is:

- Cloudy
- Brownish or grayish
- Has an odor

If you break out in a rash or get sick, you waited too long!

If you seal the drain or use a pond liner, you need to use a siphon or a transfer pump to drain your water.

If you are not using any product or technology to sanitize your water, I suggest changing it every 3-4 days or no less frequently than once per week.

If you do not bathe or rinse off before getting into your cold plunge, it is best to change your water every 3 – 4 days.

Regardless of the sanitation methods used, it is a good idea to replace your water every 3 – 6 months. Drain all of your water. Do not do partial water replacements because the water you leave in could have microorganisms in it.

■ DRAINING

CAUTION: Never lift or tilt a full chest freezer to drain it. You risk damaging the freezer and yourself. ALWAYS unplug the chest freezer and all other components before you drain it.

Drain your chest freezer for regular cleaning or if it will not be used for an extended time. There are three ways to drain your chest freezer.

Regardless of which method you use, a small amount of water will remain in the bottom. Use towels to remove this water. Another option is to gently turn the chest freezer onto its side and tilt or prop it up to create a slope for the water to drain.

Be careful when tilting or moving the chest freezer or you may damage the outside walls or the mechanics.

Built-in Drain

Most chest freezers have a built-in drain with a plug on the inside and the outside. An adapter that plugs into a standard water hose is usually included.

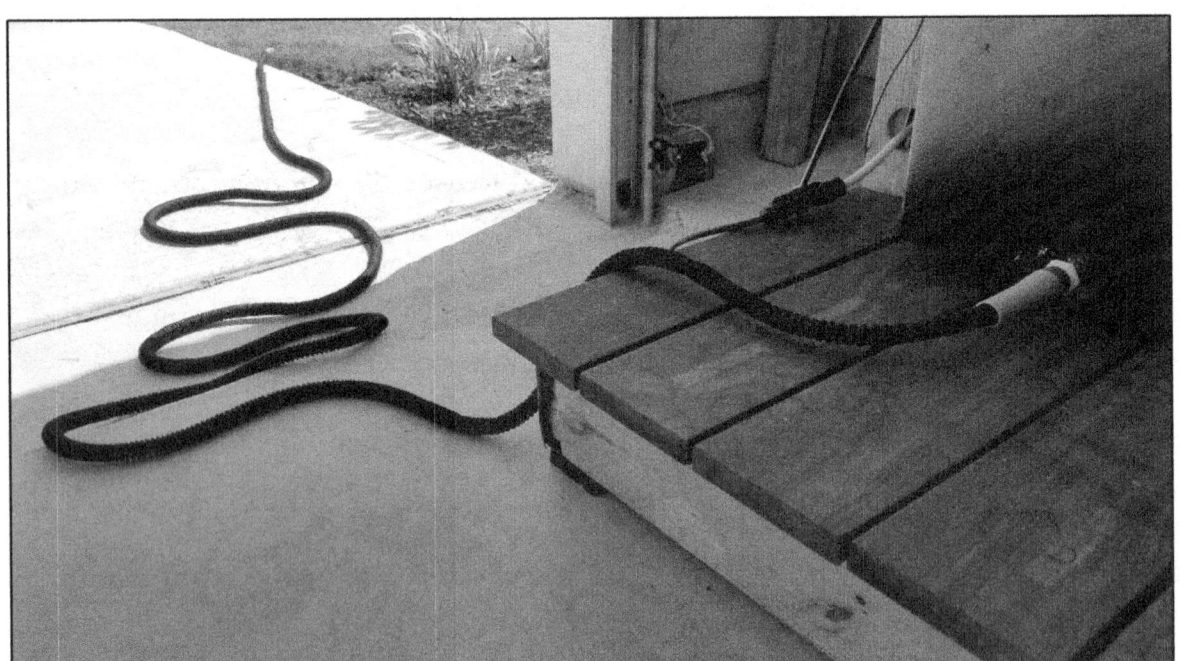

Drain adapter and garden hose

Remove the outside drain plug first. Push the hose adapter into the drain and twist to ensure a good seal. It only needs to be finger tight. Attach your garden hose and place the other end where you want the water. Then remove the inner drain plug.

Cold water should not damage your grass but may damage flowers.

It may take a while (15 – 30+ minutes) for the water to drain. If you want to speed up the process, you can use a small bucket, although this is labor-intensive.

After the water drains and you have dried the inside of the cold plunge, put the two drain plugs back in place.

Siphon

If the built-in drain has been covered or sealed, use a siphon or pump to remove the water from your cold plunge.

There are two types of siphons. The old-fashioned manual method requires a good set of lungs and a hose or tube small enough that you can create a seal around it with your mouth. It is a slow process.

Hand-crank or squeeze siphons cost between $10 - $20 and make siphoning faster.

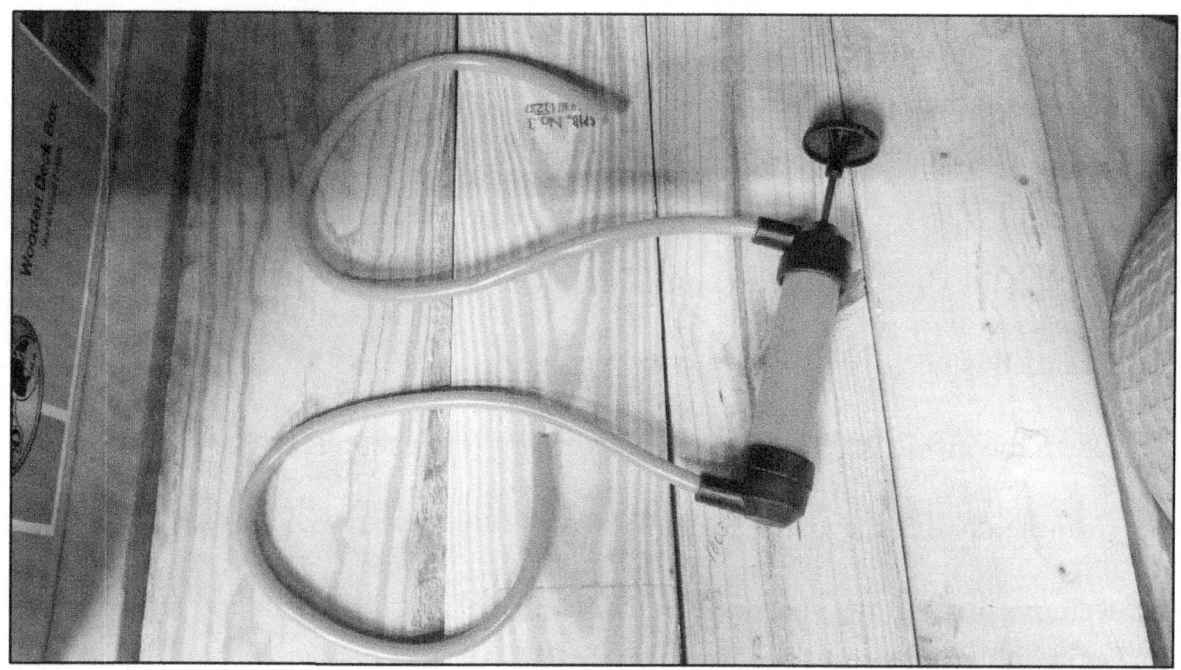

Hand pump siphon

Pump

You can use either a transfer pump or bilge pump. Using a pump is much faster than the built-in drain plug or siphoning.

Keep in mind that these pumps create pressure, so use a special pump hose for the intake. A standard garden hose may collapse or break if attached to the intake.

A standard garden hose works fine for the output of the pump.

Pumps come in two kinds: submersible and non-submersible. The submersible pumps usually leave a few inches of water, which is why I prefer the non-submersible pumps.

When you get to the last few inches of water, hold the hose underwater to drain as much as you can. If you have a liner, be sure there is no suction directly on the liner, because it may break or weaken the liner.

Watch it closely and turn it off while the hose is still underwater. Letting air into the intake hose may damage the pump.

 ## STORING YOUR CHEST FREEZER

If your cold plunge will be unused for more than a couple of weeks, it is a good idea to drain it. If you plan to be gone for an extended time, draining and storing your chest freezer helps extend its life and reduce the risk of potential accidents while you are gone.

1. Unplug the chest freezer and any components.

2. Drain all water.

3. Clean the inside walls with a mild detergent (dish soap is OK).

4. Completely dry the inside walls.

5. Remove any tubing, sensors, or other components. Dry them and store them separately (not in the chest freezer).

6. Put an open box of baking soda inside the cold plunge.

7. Turn the chest freezer so that the front is facing a wall.

8. Place a folded cloth or sponge between the top wall and lid to allow for ventilation.

9. Carefully place loose cloths or small towels around the compressor to reduce dust.

10. There is a danger of children climbing into a chest freezer and suffocating if the lid closes. If you have children, there are additional safety options:

    a. Store the chest freezer in a locked room,

    b. Place tie-down straps around it to prevent the lid from opening, or

    c. Remove the lid and set it aside, separate from the chest freezer.

Back in Action

If your cold plunge has been in storage, there are a few things to do before you put it back into use.

1. Inspect everything for damage or rust. If you find damage, call an appliance repair person.

2. Make sure that all of the wires and components are still intact

3. Carefully vacuum or wipe any dust, spider webs, bugs or other debris off of the mechanics.

4. Clean the interior with mild soap (dish detergent) and water.

REPAIRING OR REPLACING EQUIPMENT

All mechanical things eventually break down. Chest freezers, ozone generators, and UV lights have parts that eventually fail. Liners can tear or break.

Because of this, set aside a little money each month to prepare for these inevitable breakdowns. Whether your repair or replace the equipment is up to you.

Out of curiosity, I have priced replacement parts for a few different chest freezers. A new compressor can run between $200 - $300 if you do the labor yourself. If you pay an expert, it can cost between $300 - $500, which is almost as much as buying a new chest freezer.

When the cost to repair is more than half the price to buy a new one, it is generally a better idea to buy a new one.

Manufacturers built older models of chest freezers with larger motors and higher quality components. They could last 30-40 years and still work.

Newer chest freezers are built with smaller motors (to be more energy efficient) and lower-quality materials. When used for their intended purpose, new chest freezers are expected to last between 5 – 15 years.

Converting your freezer into a cold plunge adds several variables as well as wear and tear that was not planned for in the design.

We don't have enough long-term data yet to know with any certainty, but if you have correctly sealed your chest freezer and keep it clean, it is reasonable to expect it to last between 2 – 5 years. Hopefully more.

As of October 2020, we have reports of chest freezers lasting more than 4 years.

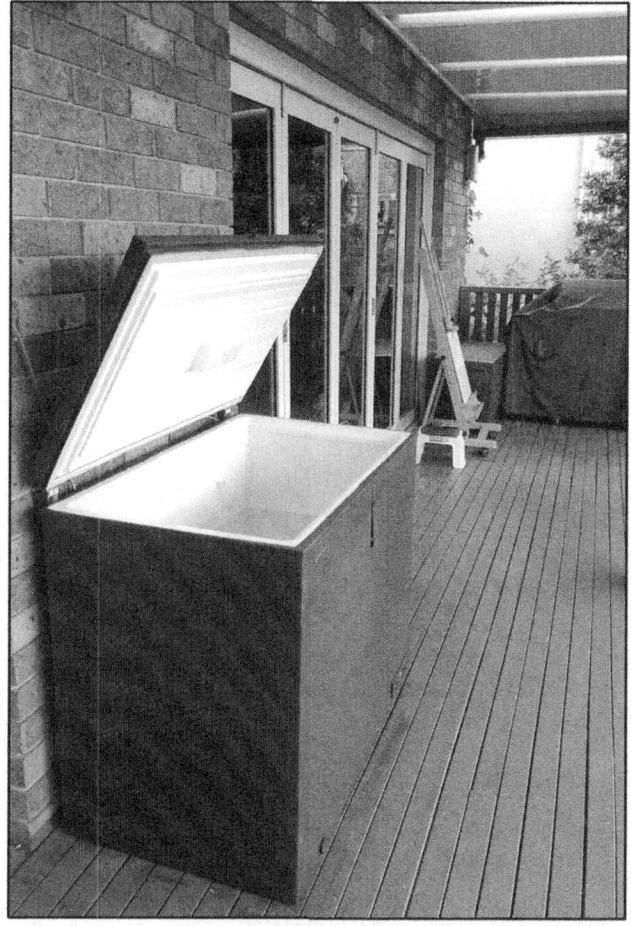

David Akers, Sydney, Australia

Brand / Size: Westinghouse 320 L (11-cu. ft.)

Location: Outdoors on a covered deck

Seams: Sealed with Selley's Knead-It Aqua

Water Sanitation: Pump/filter with built-in UV light with plans to add Epsom salts or H2O2

Inspiration for Cold Water Immersion: My motivation for cold immersion is to have tools to conjure up more energy because I'm going to need it very soon. [Editor's Note: David has two children under 5 and one on the way!] Combining the cold part of WHM* with a bunch of other health related stuff to fill my energy tank for greater physical and mental health to support my family.

*WHM = Wim Hof Method

"

*Love yourself enough to
create an environment in your life
that is conducive to the nourishment
of your personal growth.*

*Allow yourself to let go of
the people, thoughts, and situations
that poison your well-being.*

*Cultivate a vibrant surrounding and
commit yourself to making choices
that will help you release the greatest expression
of your unique beauty and purpose.*

Steve Maraboli

"

Conclusion

If you apply what you learn in this guide, you should have a new chest freezer cold plunge up and running quickly and easily. You can also expect to have fewer problems than those who had to figure out along the way what worked and what didn't.

If you have any questions, the best place to reach out to me is on the Chest Freezer Cold Plunge Facebook Group. Private messages are easy to miss.

I'd love to hear from you about how this guide has helped you as well as any suggestions or constructive criticism on how it can be improved.

Many people have sent messages about how this information has helped them save time and money or conquer their fear of getting started.

Others have let me know how finally getting a chest freezer set up has dramatically improved their health or allowed them to manage chronic pain, or prepare for athletic events and competitions. These stories are amazing and heart-warming.

If you would like to send pictures or a testimonial about your results, see Appendix N.

If you discover a new product that you'd like to recommend, please have it in use and working for at least 12 months with proven results.

Over the long haul, the more people who report back about what works and doesn't, the more this guide can be refined, saving everyone time and money.

Happy cold plunging!

"

Eustress occurs when the gap between
what one has and what one wants
is slightly pushed, but not overwhelmed.

The goal is not out of reach
but is slightly more than one can handle.

This fosters challenge and motivation
since the goal is in sight.

The function of challenge is to motivate a person
towards improvement and a goal.

Craig Smith

"

Appendices

APPENDIX A: THE BENEFITS OF COLD-WATER IMMERSION

It's beyond the scope of this guide to go into much detail about the benefits of spending time in icy water, but the bottom line is that certain kinds of stress (called positive stress, or eustress) are great for your health.

Evidence indicates that regularly plunging into cold water can reduce negative stress, improve your circulation and immunity, increase your metabolism, release a bunch of helpful feel-good chemicals in your brain, improve athletic recovery, and help with weight loss and depression.

Other benefits may include better sleep, healthier skin, and an overall better mood.

Recent research shows that cold water immersion helps your mitochondria, which are the parts of your cells that turn food into energy and break down waste.

A growing body of scientific evidence suggests that chronic diseases in the western world are diseases of the mitochondria. This includes Alzheimer's, diabetes, autoimmune, cancer, multiple sclerosis, Parkinson's, cardiovascular disease, bipolar disorder, anxiety disorder, schizophrenia, and chronic fatigue syndrome, among others.

A current hypothesis states that if you improve the health of your mitochondria, your overall health improves.

APPENDIX B: IMPERIAL & METRIC CONVERSION TABLES AND FORMULAS

These formulas include some rounding.

Temperature

Fahrenheit	Celsius
32	0.0
33	0.6
34	1.1
35	1.7
36	2.2
37	2.8
38	3.3
39	3.9
40	4.4
45	7.2
50	10.0
55	12.8
57	13.9
60	15.6
65	18.3
70	21.1
75	23.9
80	26.7

<u>Conversion Formulas</u>

Fahrenheit to Celsius

$(F - 32) \div 1.8 = C$

Example

$(40° F - 32) = 8$

$8 \times .55 = 4.4° C$

Celsius to Fahrenheit

$(C \times 1.8) + 32 = F$

Example

$(4.4° C) \times 1.8 = 7.92$

$7.92 + 32 = 39.92° F$

Volume of Water

Gallons	Liters
20	76
30	114
40	151
50	189
60	227
70	265
80	303
90	341
100	379
125	473
150	568
200	757
250	946
300	1,136

Conversion Formulas

Gallons to Liters

g x 3.78 = L

Example
(80 gallons) x 3.78 = 302 L

Liters to Gallons

L ÷ 3.78 = g

Example
(400 liters) ÷ 3.78 = 106 gallons

Weight

Pounds	Kilograms
5.0	2.3
10.0	4.5
15.0	6.8
20.0	9.1
25.0	11.4
30.0	13.6
40.0	18.2
50.0	22.7
60.0	27.3
70.0	31.8
80.0	36.4
90.0	40.9
100.0	45.5

Conversion Formulas

Pounds (lbs.) into Kilograms (kg)

lbs. ÷ 2.2 = kg

Example

(10 lbs.) ÷ 2.2 = 4.5 kg

Kilograms (kg) to pounds

Kg x 2.2) = lbs.

Example

(40 kg) x 2.2 = 88 lbs.

Chest Freezer Sizes

Chest freezer sizes are primarily used for marketing and are only an approximation of the actual capacity.

The cubic feet sizes listed in this table represent sizes available in the US. The equivalent liters are listed for reference, but may not be the actual sizes of available chest freezers available in other countries.

The approximate volume of water listed takes into consideration that the water should be filled about 6 inches below the top of the wall, and accounts for the space taken up by the cover over the compressor.

Volume of Chest Freezer	Volume of Water	Amount of Salt
7-cu. ft. / 198 L	39 gal. / 148 L	33 lbs. / 15 kg
15-cu. ft. / 424 L	75 gal. / 284 L	63 lbs. / 29 kg
21-cu. ft. / 594 L	108 gal. / 409 L	91 lbs. / 42 kg
25-cu. ft. / 708 L	179 gal. / 678 L	150 lbs. / 68 kg

Conversion Formulas

Cubic Feet to Liters

(Cu. ft.) X 28.32 = liters

Example

(7-cu. ft.) X 28.32 = 197 liters

Liters to Cubic Feet

L ÷ 28.32 = cubic feet

Example

(400 liters) ÷ 28.32 = 14-cu. ft.

APPENDIX C: HOW MUCH CRUSHED ICE IS NEEDED TO COOL WATER

If you want to do a traditional ice bath, how much ice will you need to make your water cold enough?

This formula uses Imperial measurements.

Variables:

gal = gallons of water   t1 = current temp. (in degrees Fahrenheit) of water

i = lbs. of ice   t2 = desired temp (in F) of water

Formula:

$$(gal / 1{,}000) \times (t1 - t2) \times 43.75 = i$$

Example
gal = 100 gallons of water
t1 = current water temp is 75° F
t2 = you want the water to be 40° F

$$(100 \text{ gallons} \div 1{,}000) \times (75 - 40) \times 43.75 = i$$

$$(.1) \times (35) \times 43.75 = i$$

$$3.5 \times 43.75 = i$$

$$153.125 = i$$

> ## PRO TIP
> Adding enough salt to your water lowers the freezing point, and reduces the amount of ice needed. See Chapter 14, Breaking the Ice: Prevention

Metric Formula: This has been derived from the imperial formula and will get you pretty close, but may not be exact.

$$(\text{Liters} \div 4000) \times (t1 - t2) \times 38 = \text{kg of ice needed}$$

APPENDIX D: MAJOR CHEST FREEZER BRANDS

There are too many countries for this list to be inclusive. However, here are some of the major brands found in a few different parts of the world:

Australia	Europe	USA
Hisense	Bosch	Amana
Haier	BEKO	Frigidaire
Westinghouse,	Haier	GE
Fisher & Paykel	Kenwood	Kenmore
	LEC	Maytag
	Miele	Magic Chef
		Whirlpool

APPENDIX E: TEMPERATURE CONTROLLERS

Here are a few recommended temperature controllers. Be sure to get one that works with the voltage in your country.

AquaLogic NEMA 4, Single Stage Controller, 115 v - $137

AquaLogic, 230V - $158

Inkbird ITC-308 Max.1200W Heater, Cool Device Temperature Controller - $35

WILLHI WH1436A Temperature Controller - $29.99

APPENDIX F: SEALANTS AND LINERS

Sealants

Method	Cost	Installation	Longevity/Notes	Recommended
JB Water Weld (12 - 20 tubes)	$60 - $140	Simple, but time-consuming. Putty must be thoroughly mixed.	Likely to outlast your chest freezer.	Yes – first choice!
100% Pure Silicone (2 - 4 tubes) Use Momentive RTV103-300 ml	$34 - $80 + caulking gun	Simple and fast	Short term. Might last long term with the right product, correct prep, and application.	No / Yes General silicones are not recommended by manufacturers for continuous submerged use, but aquarium owners say the premium brands work well for large tanks.

Removable Liners

Method	Cost	Installation	Longevity/Notes	Recommended
Seamless Pond Liner (15′ x 20′) (45 mm EDPM)	$250 - $300	Simple but may take some work to fold it properly into the chest freezer	Long if used gently to prevent punctures	Yes Check compatibility with sanitation devices and chemicals.
Custom PVC Liner	$400 - $500	Simple	Unknown. Cracks and leaks may develop over time at the seams.	Maybe Check compatibility with sanitation devices and chemicals.

Method	Cost	Installation	Longevity/Notes	Recommended
Spray Liners- Do-it-yourself	$300 - $500	Complex and time-consuming. All paint must be stripped first.	Unknown. Polyethylene has good compatibility with ozone in water, but only fair compatibility in air.	Yes, unless using ozone.
Spray Liners – Professionally applied	$800 - $2,000	Easy – they do all of the prep	Unknown. Long. These liners are extremely durable. The compatibility of polyurea with ozone is unknown.	Yes, unless using ozone. If using ozone, a top-end liner will work. Check with the dealer.
Epoxy Paint	$400 - $800	Chemicals must be mixed correctly, and timing is critical.	Short. Most epoxy paints end up flaking and peeling. They can take a long time to off-gas. If the right kind of marine epoxy is used, with correct preparation and expert workmanship, it may last a very long time.	No- if you have never worked with epoxy. Yes- if you have the right kind of epoxy (VOC-free) and a very experienced person to apply / install it.

Permanent Liners

Method	Cost	Installation	Longevity/Notes	Recommended
Liquid Rubber	$200 - $400	Easy	Short – not recommended. Cold water causes rubber to crack. Not compatible with ozone. Many complaints on pool and spa forums.	No
Fiberglass	$500 - $900	Do it yourself: complex Hire a professional: easy	Long. This is the stuff used by professionals to repair holes in boats.	Maybe (No real-world data yet, but could be promising)

APPENDIX G: SANITATION METHODS

Additives

Method	Cost	Pros	Cons	Recommended
Nothing-drain and refill as needed	Your time	Simple and easy.	Wasted water. Number of off-days while water is chilled.	Yes
Standard Pool Chemicals (chlorine, acid, etc.)	Unknown	Easily available	Expensive over time. Water must be kept in balance. Bad for your skin. May be toxic.	No
Floating Spa Chemical Dispenser (chlorine or bromine only)	Less than $20 per year	Easily available	Dry skin. May bleach hair and swimsuits. Chemical sensitivities.	Yes – if you are OK with chlorine.
Epsom Salts	$30 - $50 if using farm-grade	Good for your skin. Reduces/prevents ice build-up due to lowered freezing point.	Will cause rust if splashed on exposed metal. Can get expensive over time.	Yes
Hydrogen Peroxide (35% food grade)	~ $20 for 16 ounces	Excellent for sanitation.	Dangerous if splashed onto skin or into eyes. Can get expensive over time.	Yes, if you are careful.

Devices

Method	Cost	Pros	Cons	Recommended
Pump / Filter - External	$150 - $400 + plumbing	Filters sediment. Prevents ice buildup.	Heat gain in system. Priming the pump. Condensation.	No
Pump / Filter - Submersible	$50 - $120	Filters sediment. Prevents ice buildup. Needed if ozone, UV, or pool chemicals are used.	Power cord placed over edge of freezer wall and may interfere with seal. Power cord placed through lid requires a large hole. Takes up space inside the chest freezer.	Yes
Ozone Generator - Stand-alone external unit with built-in pump	$150- $300	Superior for sanitation.	Ozone tube placed over edge of wall interferes with seal on lid. Optional tube placement requires drilling a hole in the lid. No way to test sanitation.	Yes
UV Light	$100 - $300	May have built-in aquarium pump/filter.	Bulbs are fragile and need to be replaced every 6-12 months. No way to test sanitation.	Yes

APPENDIX H: TEMPERATURE CONTROL METHODS

There are four ways to keep your water cold and reduce ice build-up.

Method	Cost	Pros	Cons
Manually Unplug and Plug-in Daily	Your time	Inexpensive.	Wasted time. If you forget you may end up with a lot of ice, or a solid block of ice, or warm water. May end up with higher energy usage/utility bills.
Heavy-Duty Mechanical Timer	$15 - $25	Mostly set and forget. Can be set to run during times when the cost of electricity is less.	Clock time is incorrect because of unplugging. Does not account for ambient temperatures, which can result in too much or not enough cooling. May need to be adjusted frequently.
Heavy Duty Digital Timer (Smart House tech)	$100 - $300	Can be programmed via smart-phone / web browser. Time resets automatically after electricity has been off.	Does not account for ambient temperatures, which can result in too much or not enough cooling. Depending on the system installed, may cause problems for those with EMF sensitivities.
Temperature Controller (Digital)	$35 - $175	Very precise. A high and low range can be set.	Sensor must be in the water, which requires a cable to be placed over the edge of the wall, which may interfere with the seal.

APPENDIX I: OZONE COMPATIBILITY

This chart is compiled from various industry sources. The following grades are a combination of the theoretical rating where no ozone concentration was given.

The rating given to JB Water Weld is from the manufacturer.

Rating Scale

    A – Excellent. No effect.

    B - Good: Minor Effect, slight corrosion, or discoloration.

    C - Fair: Moderate Effect, not recommended for continuous use. Softening or loss of strength and swelling may occur.

    D - Severe Effect: Not recommended for any use.

    E - Information not available.

Aluminum	C
EPDM	A
JB Water Weld	A
Neoprene	B
Polyethylene	In water: B In air: C
Polyurethane	A
PVC	F
Rubber	F
Silicone	A
Stainless Steel	B / C
Vinyl	B

APPENDIX J: CHEMICAL COMPATIBILITY

It is difficult to make a simple chart that lists the compatibility between various sanitation chemicals and materials used in chest freezers. A few common combinations are listed below.

If your material and chemical are not listed below, check out this website:

https://www.coleparmer.com/chemical-resistance

Rating Scale

    A – Excellent. No effect.

    B - Good: Minor Effect, slight corrosion, or discoloration.

    C - Fair: Moderate Effect, not recommended for continuous use. Softening or loss of strength and swelling may occur.

    D - Severe Effect: Not recommended for any use.

    E - Information not available.

Variables that influence chemical compatibility include temperature, pressure, concentrations, and duration of exposure.

JBWW = JB Water Weld. Selleys is comparable.

Chemical	Material						
	Aluminum	EPDM	JBWW	Polyurethane	PVC	Rubber	Silicone
Bromine	D	D	A	D	C	D	D
Chlorine	D	C	A	E	A	C	D
Epsom Salts	B	A	A	D	A	B	A
H2O2	A	A	A	B	A	B	A
NaCl (Salt)	B	A	A	D	A	A	A

APPENDIX K: DEVICE MANUFACTURERS

AquaLogic Temperature Controller

https://www.aqualogicinc.com

9558 Camino Ruiz, San Diego, CA 92126

Phone **858-292-4773**

E-mail **info@Aqualogicinc.com**

JB Water Weld

(903) 885-7696

Sulpher Springs, TX

https://www.jbweld.com/

JED Engineering

The JED 203:

Phone: (619) 401-8770

https://www.jedengineering.com   sales@jedengineering.com

APPENDIX L: BUYER'S CHECK LISTS

Used Chest Freezer Inspection Check List

General Questions

❑ Can you save money to buy a new chest freezer in the next 3-6 months? If yes, then buy a new one!

❑ How old is it?   < 5 years =OK   > 5 years = Avoid (unless free!)

❑ Temperature check. Ask the owner to plug it in 24 hours before you plan to inspect it. Bring a thermometer and place it inside for a minute or two. It should be close to 32 F (0 C)

Exterior

❑ Rust-free

❑ No huge dents or scratches

❑ No signs of damage or neglect

❑ Compressor area free of dirt, dust, and rust (unscrew panel if needed)

❑ Open and close the lid a few times

　　❑ Easy　　　　　　　　　❑ Hinges hold the lid firmly open

　　❑ Lid in fully open position is reachable from front of chest freezer

Interior

❑ Look at the inside walls, plastic molding on the tops of the walls, and the seams. Make sure that there are no cracks or splits in the paint or metal

❑ Inside lid is free of cracks and secured to the chest freezer (not loose)

❑ Make sure that there are no gaps larger than 1/4-inch (6.3 mm) between the seams of the interior walls. All seams should have small gaps or be tightly overlapped.

❑ No rust and no mold

❑ If there is a light, does it work?

❑ Inspect the seals around the lid and ensure that they are soft and pliable and not hard or missing

❑ The lock works

❑ The key is included

Exterior

❑ If there is any damage to the box or packing crate, take pictures.

❑ Look at all of the exterior walls. They should be free of dents, scratches, and signs of being dropped or damaged.

❑ Inspect handles and plastic covers over the mechanics compartment to ensure they are intact and secured to the freezer

❑ Check out the compressor. It should be free of rust and securely attached to the frame.

❑ Lift or tilt the edge of the chest freezer that has the compressor to the back and side. Listen for sounds of rattling or loose parts.

❑ Does the lid open and close easily?

❑ Is the key is included, and does the lock work?

Interior

❑ The inside walls and under the lid should be free from dents and scratches.

❑ The light (if included) should work when the lid is open and close when the lid is off

❑ Make sure that there are no gaps larger than 1/4-inch (6.3 mm) between the seams of the interior walls. All seams should have small gaps or be tightly overlapped.

Chill Test

❑ Plug in the chest freezer to a power outlet. Put a thermometer on the floor inside and close and lock the lid. Turn the dial to the coldest setting and let it run for 24-48 hours. The inside should reach 0°F (-17.7° C).

❑ Listen to the compressor when it starts working. There may be an initial rattle as it starts, but after that, it should be a quiet hum. If it is making an unusual noise or sounds loud, there may be a problem.

APPENDIX M: MAINTENANCE LOG

Brand:_____   Date Purchased:_____

Model #:_____   Serial #:_____

Date	Temp.	Notes

APPENDIX N: TRAINING LOG

Date	Temp.	Duration	Notes

APPENDIX O: RESOURCES

Here are helpful resources to learn more about the benefits of cold training.

Online Training & Live Classes

Wim Hof Method   www.WimHofMethod.com

Dr. Jack Kruze (MD)   www.JackKruse.com

Books

What Doesn't Kill Us: How Freezing Water, Extreme Altitude, and Environmental Conditioning Will Renew Our Lost Evolutionary Strength

By Scott Carney

Health & Fitness

Dr. Rhonda Patrick

www.foundmyfitness.com

APPENDIX P: TELL US ABOUT YOUR SETUP

Sending in details about your setup adds to the body of research and helps improve the recommendations in this guide. On top of that, it is exciting to find out what setup you have chosen and how it helps you. Include as much of the following info as you can.

Pictures
Please use landscape mode (widescreen) and a high-resolution setting.

Your setup:
1. What is your full name?

2. Is it ok to include your name in future editions or do you prefer to be anonymous?

3. In what country do you live?

4. What brand and size of chest freezer do you have?

5. Where do you keep it (inside, garage, covered porch, etc.)?

6. Did you seal the seams? If yes, what type of sealant did you use?

7. Do you have a liner in your chest freezer? If yes, provide details about the materials, if it was custom-made, etc.

8. What is your average water temperature?

9. How long do you spend in the water at that temperature?

10. How often do you get into your chest freezer cold plunge?

11. How do you control the water temperature (manually unplug/plug in, timer, controller)?

12. What water sanitation methods do you use (if any)?

13. How often do you change the water?

14. How long have you had this setup running?

15. What issues or problems have you experienced?

16. Why do you do cold water immersion?

17. Have you participated in any online or live Wim Hof Method courses? If yes, which ones and when?

18. In what ways has this guide been helpful to you?

Send your answers to: to coldinfo@johnrichter.com

Notes

_____

_____

_____

_____

_____

_____

_____

_____

_____

_____

_____

APPENDIX Q: FAQ

These are the most Frequently Asked Questions on the Chest Freezer Cold Plunge Facebook group.

Top Mistakes to Avoid

1. **Buying a chest freezer with bare aluminum walls.**

   The insides of chest freezers are either bare aluminum or painted metal. The aluminum walls and floors are thin and are easily dented and damaged, causing leaks. Aluminum (and impurities in the aluminum) can react badly to various sanitation methods. Spend the extra money to get a chest freezer with the interior painted by the manufacturer.

2. **Not sealing the seams.**

   Chest freezers are not waterproof. If you don't seal the seams correctly, water will get inside the walls. This causes rust and mold, makes your chest freezer work harder than it has to, and greatly reduces the life of the compressor.

3. **Incorrectly sealing the seams.**

   The idea of "Penny-wise and pound foolish" applies here. In order to save a bit of money now, people use cheap, inferior, or untested products to seal the seams. Few people will admit that this is a seriously bad idea until they get a bunch of rust coming out of their seams. Then they have wasted money and time and added frustration.

   Stick with recommended products that have proven to work over time.

4. **Not supporting the bottom of the chest freezer.**

   When you fill up the chest freezer with water, it adds several hundreds of pounds (kg) of weight. It also adds pressure to the walls and floors in a way that it was not designed to support. To help your chest freezer support this weight, place several shims between the feet on the outside bottoms of the freezer.

Safety

1. **How do I keep from being electrocuted?**

   Unplug the chest freezer and all other devices before you get in. Don't use a phone or wear headphones while in the water. Make sure your hands and feet are dry before you plug everything back in. Make sure you have a GFCI outlet. Keep all other electrical cords devices and tools away from your chest freezer area where they could get wet.

2. **Do I need a ground fault circuit interrupt (GFCI) outlet?**

   Yes. If you don't have one, buy a GFCI extension cord.

3. **I heard there is a capacitor in the chest freezer that still holds a charge even after it is unplugged. Doesn't this create a risk for shock?**

   The appliance repairmen who responded to this question said that most chest freezers do not have capacitors in them. An electrician reported that even if there is a capacitor in your chest freezer, it would be unlikely to cause electrical shock, and if it did, the shock would not be strong enough to cause serious harm.

4. **How do I keep from getting locked inside?**

   New chest freezers, by law, have lids that do not lock automatically. If you are looking at used chest freezers, do not buy one that automatically locks. Be kind to your spouse, partner, children and roommates.

5. **What about child safety?**

   Chest freezers create an air-tight seal when the lid is closed. Small children can get trapped inside and suffocate. The walls can get hot which can cause minor burns. Ice water can be deadly for children (and adults) who are not trained. Do NOT let children play in or around your chest freezer or use it without adult supervision.

6. **How do I modify the freezer lid so it stays open without crashing down on my head?**

   Most new chest freezers have hinges that are strong enough to stay open on their own. If your lid does not stay open, you can replace the hinges, which are expensive. A simple option is to place a towel on the top of the wall, which would prevent the lid from closing. Another option is to connect an eyebolt to the top of the lid and to the wall with a short piece of rope, cord, or cable between them. The eyebolt must go all the way through the lid and have a washer and nut inside to keep it in place. Use a carabiner or quick disconnect on the cord to make it easy to adjust and remove.

7. **The outside of my chest freezer is very hot. Is that normal?**

Yes. Make sure you have enough space around the chest freezer for ventilation. Keep children and pets away.

8. **What are VOCs?**

Volatile Organic Chemicals, which can cause serious health issues. Do not use any product with VOCs because they could leach into your water and potentially cause long term health issue.

9. **Is it OK to use products labelled as "food grade"?**

In the US, the Food and Drug Administration (FDA) uses the term "food grade" to indicate that a product is safe to use around food. That does not necessarily mean that the product is suitable for long-term use under water. It also does not necessarily mean it is the highest grade available.

Buying / Shopping / Research

1. **What size of chest freezer do I need?**

Get a size that feels comfortable. 14 cu. ft. (400 L) seem to be a good baseline. If you are taller than 5'10 or weigh more than 200 lbs. (91 kg), a larger freezer might be better.

2. **Do I have to sit in a freezer before purchasing?**

No, but it can help you figure out what size is best for you. If you don't have one that you can sit in, get the internal measurements and mock up a chest freezer using the corner of a room and some tape, boxes, chairs, or whatever is handy. This will give you a feel for the size. Be sure to include the area over the compressor.

3. **What is the absolute minimal I need to do for converting my chest freezer into a cold plunge?**

Waterproof the seams.

---

4. **Which is better, painted or unpainted?**

   Chest freezers with interiors painted by the manufacturer are more durable and have fewer problems. I only recommend unpainted chest freezers if you do not have the money to buy a new chest freezer with a painted interior.

5. **Should I buy a new or used chest freezer?**

   If it is in your budget, new is better. If it will take more than 6 months to save for a new chest freezer, buy a used one so you can at least get started. Be advised that used chest freezers can die unexpected and have a number of problems that may not be obvious at first. Prepare for the possibility of extra work and frustration. In my opinion, it is better to delay gratification, and save to buy a new one. It will be worth it!

6. **Which brand / manufacturer is the best?**

   For our purpose there is not much difference. Stick to major brands that have good reviews online.

7. **Where is the best location for my chest freezer?**

   Find a spot that is convenient, and protects your chest freezer from the elements. Some good places are: covered porch, garage, sunroom, and basement. The more you can protect your chest freezer from sun, rain, hail, critters, humidity, and big temperature changes, the better.

8. **Is it OK to put my chest freezer on a second floor porch / patio / room?**

   Load bearing calculations are complex and best left to structural engineers. Most floors can hold fish aquariums that hold less than 100 gallons of water. If you have a chest freezer that is smaller than 15 cu. ft. (425 L) it *should* be OK. If you have a larger chest freezer, it should be placed on the ground floor or on a concrete slab. Every building is different. It is strongly advisable to consult a structural engineer.

9. **I live in an apartment. Can I set up a chest freezer?**

   Yes, and… read your lease agreement, which may forbid fish aquariums over a certain size. While the chest freezer is not technically an aquarium, they might find you in violation of your lease. If you are not on the ground floor see

Question 8, above. Also most insurance policies do not cover water issues and you could be held liable if there is damage due to leaks.

10. **I live in an apartment. How do I fill and drain my chest freezer?**

    To fill your chest freezer, use a faucet to garden hose adapter. A transfer pump can be used to fill/drain water from/to the bathtub. A siphon can be used to drain the water. Run the hose outside to the balcony/porch or to a sink, shower, or bathtub.

Waterproofing

1. **Does the freezer need to be completely sealed?**

   Yes. Seal all seams, including the upper seam around the plastic molding on top of the walls.

2. **Several people have posted that they just filled up their chest freezer with water and did not seal the seams and it is working fine.**

   Yeah, I did that too. It only took 3 days for rust to seep out of the seams. On some freezers it takes longer. However, eventually water will damage the insides of the walls beyond repair. This greatly shortens the life of the chest freezer.

3. **How do I seal it?**

   Epoxy putty. However, you need to use the right product. JB Water Weld or Selleys Knead-it Aqua are good epoxies that come in an easy-to-use putty.

4. **What about silicone?**

   Use at your own risk. A *few* people have reported good results over time using silicone. However, the largest number of leaks and rust problems have also been reported by those who used silicone. If you are going to use silicone, you must properly prepare and clean the surface, use a high-quality product, correctly apply it, and let it cure long enough. If you insist on using silicone, go with a product used by aquarium builders: Momentive 100 series in the 300 ml tubes that go into a standard caulking gun. My advice? Spend the extra money to buy JB Water Weld (or comparable product) – it's worth it.

5. **How do I correctly apply silicone?**

   If you insist on using silicone, watch a few handyman videos on YouTube to get this info. Again, the odds are against you. I still recommend JB Water Weld.

6. **What products should be *not* be used to seal the seams?**

   Cheap caulking or silicone, marine tape, paint-on rubber, blu tack, liquid rubber, rubberized paint, Rust-Oleum, FlexSeal and chewing gum. None of the products are meant for prolonged underwater use. Some are toxic. Read on for recommended products.

7. **What products can I use to seal the seams?**

   JB Water Weld (or a comparable 2-part epoxy putty) is still my top recommendation. Custom pool liners and professionally applied VOC-free spray liners such as the Platinum Line-X product have promise.

8. **JB Water Weld is not available (or 3-4x the cost) in my country. Is there an alternative?**

   Yes. Selleys Knead-It Aqua is good. If you can't find either one, look for a 2-part epoxy putty. That said, if you can't find a comparable product, spend the extra money anyway. The time and frustration you will save by sealing the seams correctly will be worth it.

9. **If I install a liner, do I still need to seal the seams?**

   Yes. If (when) the liner cracks, breaks, or leaks, you will be glad that you sealed the seams.

10. **If I seal the seams do I need to use a liner?**

    No, but it can extend the life of your chest freezer. Liners are strongly recommended if you have bare aluminum walls.

11. **What kind of liner should I get?**

    There are two types of liners: removable and permanent. Pond liners are removable. Liners that need to be sprayed or painted on are permanent.

12. **What is the best pond liner?**

    It depends on your plan for water sanitation. Chorine, salt, UV light, and ozone can discolor or deteriorate certain types of plastics. Be sure to check material compatibility. If your sanitation plan is to drain, clean, a refill your water without additives or devices EPDM is a good choice of material. The thickness of the liner also makes a difference. 45 mils (1.14 mm) is a good choice.

13. **What is the best permanent liner?**

    Professionally applied liners are the best. Top-tier products from Line-X and Rhino are resistant to chemicals, ozone and UV and will not leach VOCs into your water. We are starting to get good reports from people using two-part marine epoxy. However, these types of liners can require labor intensive preparation to the inside of your chest freezer, including stripping all of the existing paint. The also require impeccable timing, meticulous measuring and mixing, and careful application. These Do-It-Yourself (DIY) liners are only recommended for people with moderate to high levels of skill.

14. **What else can you tell me about professionally applied truck bed liners like Line-**X?

    If you decide to go with one of these products, you might need to make a bunch of calls to different franchise owners to find one who will apply the product to a chest freezer.

    Go with the top tier product. With Line-X, this would be the Platinum version.

    We do not yet know how these products will impact the ability of your chest freezer to chill the water. While these products have no insulative properties, they may cause your chest freezer to work harder, which could reduce the life of the compressor. So far, we know of one person who reported about a month of success so far with his Line-X freezer.

15. **How do you mix JB Water Weld?**

    It needs to be hand-mixed, just a little at a time. There are two materials in the stick of putty. One is white and the other is gray. Mix, roll, and squish them together until they blend completely into an off-white color.

16. **How do you apply JB Water Weld?**

    Once mixed, roll it into a ball. Then roll the ball into a little snake. Push the snake into the seams. The line of putty over the seam should be about 1" (2.5 cm) wide, and about 1/8" (.3 cm) thick.

17. **How much JB Water Weld does it take to seal a chest freezer?**

    Different brands and sizes have different lengths of seams. One tube of JB Water weld covers about 16 inches (40.6 cm) of seams. It will take 15 – 20 tubes to seal a Whirlpool 14 cu. ft. (424 L) chest freezer, not including the seam at the top wall and trim.

18. **How long does it take to apply JB Water Weld to all of the seams?**

It depends on the size of the freezer and how fast you work. With two people working at a steady, but friendly pace, one person mixing and the other applying, it will take about 5-6 hours.

19. **Are there any issues or concerns with using JB Water Weld?**

Yes. You must completely mix the two different compounds for it to cure. You must correctly prepare and clean the surface. Follow the directions on the package. Work in a well-ventilated area.

20. **You seem to recommend JB Water Weld a lot – do you get kickbacks from that company?**

No, but it would be nice!

21. **Do I need to seal the drain?**

The hole in the drain? Generally, no. If it leaks after you fill it, make sure the plugs are secure. If there is a piece of plastic that the drain plug goes into, seal the seam around the outer edge of that piece of plastic and the floor.

22. **Can I use silicone for the seals?**

Yes, but again we are having a lot of reports of problems. If you insist on using silicone, to increase your odds of good results, use a product recommended by people who build large fish aquariums. The Momentive RTV 100-series is best. However, even with this product, we have had reports of problems.

23. **How does JB Water Weld compare to Momentive RTV Silicone?**

Both products are safe in water after curing (no toxic chemicals) and stand up to cold, chlorine, salt, UV light, ozone, and H_2O_2. Both require the surface to be prepared.

JBWW needs to be mixed thoroughly or it will not cure. If not mixed correctly it needs to be removed and done again with new putty.

Silicone does not need to be mixed. It can be applied with a standard caulking gun.

Silicone relies on moisture and humidity in the air to cure properly, which could be another potential issue. JBWW cures by chemical reaction, which is one reason why it is significantly stronger.

I have seen several posts from people who have sealed their chest freezer using silicone, and they still got rust. I have seen zero reports of rust after correctly applying JBWW.

This may have been an issue with not preparing the surface correctly or poor workmanship, and not the silicone itself.

The high-quality silicone (Momentive RTV 100 series) is less expensive than JBWW.

JB Water Weld will fully cure in 24 hours. It is best to let the silicone cure for at least 7-10 days.

There are *far* more problems reported with silicone (including the Momentive brand) than with JB Water Weld.

I feel more comfortable if the seams have been sealed with JB Water Weld.

24. **How long does it take for the smell to go away?**
JB Water Weld typically has no odor after 24 hours. Silicone might take up to a week. Other products (like some epoxy resin paints) might take months. Temporary liners might take days, weeks, or months. The top-tier professionally applied liners like Rhino and Line-X are VOC-free should be odor free within 24 hours. Their lower-tier products may off-gas indefinitely.

Water Sanitation

1. **Depending on my level of sanitation, how long will the water stay clean?**
    There are many variables. Anywhere from 3 days up to 6 months.

2. **Can I use pool chemicals to keep my water clean?**
    Yes, but keep it simple. Use a floating chemical dispenser with tablets. Change out the water every 1 – 3 months.

3. **What is the most economic filter?**
    Filters need to be used with a pump. Find a submersible aquarium pump with a built-in filter. The flow rate should be 2-3 times the volume of water.

4. **What is the most economic and easy sanitation without chemicals?**
    Shower or rinse every time before getting in. Completely drain and clean your freezer every 3 – 7 days. Refill with fresh water.

5. **What is the difference between ozone and UV?**
    The main difference is that ozone kills bacteria, viruses, mold, and fungus. UV disrupts the DNA, preventing microorganisms from reproducing.

6. **Which one is better, ozone or UV?**
    Both are valid methods of sanitizing water. There are a lot of details that must be right for UV to sanitize the water. For that reason, I prefer ozone.

7. **Doesn't using an ozone generator hurt the environment?**
    No. The only byproduct of using ozone to sanitize your water is oxygen.

8. **What kind of ozone generator should I get?**
    You need one with a built-in pump. The ones meant for spas / hot tubs will not work. Make sure to order a product that works with the electrical requirements in your country.
    High end: JED 203
    Low end: A2Z Aqua-6 or Aqua-8

9. **I've seen many posts from people using cheap UV lights saying that their water is clean. What is the problem with UV?**
    UV light can do one of two things: clarify or sanitize, and there is a significant

difference between them. When the water is clarified, it is only made clear, but that does not deactivate harmful microorganisms. Only sanitizing will do that. Most of these people have water that looks clean, but could be full of bacteria.

10. **How do I choose a good UV filter that will work?**

There is a very detailed answer to this question. The best website I have found to completely answer that question is linked below. For a 15 cu. ft. (400 L) chest freezer you need two of these models: SunSUN CUP 13 Watt UV pump/filters. One on each end of your tub. The only other tricky part is that you have to find a way to slow down the output, which means half-way blocking where the water comes out. Cheaper SunSUN- and other brand's- models are not recommended.

http://www.americanaquariumproducts.com

11. **Can I use hydrogen peroxide (H2O2) to sanitize my water?**

Yes. You must use 35% food grade H2O2. Refer to the chapters on water sanitation for details.

Pump/ Filter

1. **What kind of pump should I use?**

Use a submersible aquarium, pond, or fountain pump with a built-in filter. The flow rate should be 2-3 times the volume of your water. 3x is better. 4x might be too much.

2. **How do I connect the pump to the freezer for filtering?**

The pump sits inside the freezer, underwater. The power cord is run out of the freezer between the lid and the top of the wall.

3. **Is it OK to use an external pump?**

Yes, but you might have some problems.

- Additional work is needed to plumb the intake and return lines through the lid of the chest freezer.

- You may get a lot of condensation on the pump and plumbing. Insulation may help. -Heat-gain from the ambient air can cause your water temperature to be warmer than desired, and result in your chest freezer running more often than it should (which reduces the lifespan of the compressor).

4. **How long does the filtration pump need to run per cold water plunge?**

   Pump/filters are meant to be run 24/7. Putting them on a timer will make the motor start and stop frequently, which can reduce the lifespan.

Using the Cold Plunge

1. **How do I keep the freezer lid sealed?**

   Lock it after each use. If you have cables or wires running between the seal, cut some weather stripping or foam rubber sealant to place around it. Do not use spray foam. Many people do not add any kind insulation to the cables and wires and it seems to work just fine without.

2. **How do I break the ice without hurting the walls?**

   Only hit the ice 2-3 inches (5-8 cm) away from the wall. Do not use anything made of metal. Plastic, rubber, or PVC is better. It is safer for you and the chest freezer to avoid ice buildup.

3. **Ice / frost is building up on the walls. Should I scrape it off?**

   No. Chipping or scraping the ice risks damaging the walls or the chiller coils inside the walls. Manufacturers recommend defrosting your chest freezer when 1/4" (.64 cm) of ice builds up on the walls. Use can use water to melt the ice, or drain, dry and clean the chest freezer.

Keeping the Water Cold

1. **How cold should the water be?**

   There are many ways to enjoy cold water immersion. There are benefits starting as warm as 57° F (13.8° C). Do not go any colder than 32° F (0° C).

2. **How long does it take to chill the water?**

   There are many variables at play. Plan for 2 -5 days.

3. **Do I have to use a temperature controller?**

   No. Just unplug and plug it in as needed. Keep a close eye on it, however. If you wait too long to plug it back in, you'll have warm water. If you wait too long to unplug it you could have a thick block of ice to break through. You can also use an appliance timer. However, temperature controllers will take out the guesswork and make your life a lot easier.

4. **What temperature controller should I use?**

   Here are two recommendations.

   High end: AquaLogic Nema 4 Single Stage Controller. $160

   Less expensive: Inkbird ITC-308 Max. $30 - $35

5. **How do I set up the temperature controller with a pump/filter to prevent ice build-up?**

   Even with a temperature controller, ice will still form. Installing a submersible pump/filter will keep the water circulating and reduce or eliminate ice build-up.

6. **Considering running costs, how low should I keep the water temp?**

   There is not much of a difference in operating costs between various temperatures. Use the temperature that works best for your purpose.

Cold Training

1. **I'm new, what do you recommend?**

   Get training. Watching a bunch of free videos on YouTube is not a substitute for training from people who know what they are doing.

2. **How long should I stay in the water?**

   This depends on the temperature, your goals, and your body. Wim Hof Method trainers recommend working up to 2 – 5 minutes in water under 40 F (4.4 C). However, you can stay in until you start to shiver, feel burning, or pins and needles. Pay attention to your body.

3. **How do I know that this cold therapy is doing anything besides run up my electric bill?**

   How do you feel afterward? That is the short-term answer. Long term? There is a growing body of research showing the benefits of cold-water immersion.

   Check out the resources section in Appendix O.

   Also check out this page on the Wim Hof website:

   https://www.wimhofmethod.com/science

There are hundreds of posts on the Wim Hof Method Facebook group from people who have received amazing or life changing improvements from combining cold water exposure with the breathing method taught by Wim. Until we have hard science on the specifics about length of immersion at different temperatures, you'll just have to be willing to trust your body and be ahead of the science.

Notes

" *There is something wonderfully*

bold and liberating about saying yes

to our entire imperfect and messy life. "

Tara Brach

About the Author

John Richter lives in Austin, Texas with his daughter, Natalia. He has a passion for figuring things out, teaching, and transformation.

John is available for consultations via phone and Skype and might be available to help you convert your chest freezer in person.

For more information, contact John on the Chest Freezer Cold Plunge Facebook group or send an email to coldinfo@johnrichter.com.

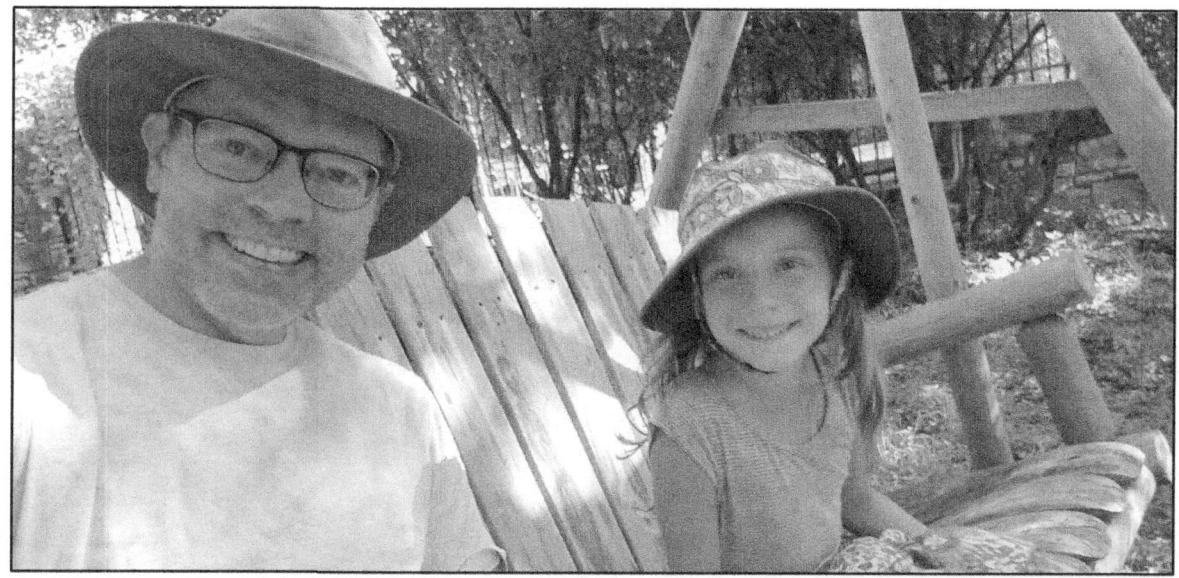

John and his daughter, Natalia

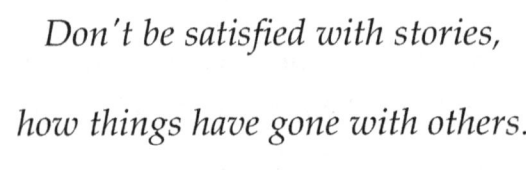

Don't be satisfied with stories,

how things have gone with others.

Unfold your own myth.

Rumi

Made in the USA
Monee, IL
28 March 2023